The
EVERYTHING
Low-Salt Cookbook

Dear Reader:

Salt is an essential part of our diets. It's too much salt that can be a problem—especially for salt-sensitive individuals. Thus, my goal in this book is to help you find ways to get your salt consumption under control.

Few recipes in this book suggest adding salt to the recipe. I find it best to use a little gray sea salt to season dishes to my taste once I've cooked them. I'm not a big fan of salty foods, so it seldom takes more than a pinch of that gray sea salt to season a dish to my liking. Granted, there are exceptions. But even with those exceptions, I think you'll be amazed at how little salt is needed to enhance the flavor of good food.

By employing some food fixin' tricks that you'll discover throughout the book, it's easy to fix flavorful food. When you employ those tricks, even if you do feel the need to salt your food at the table, it takes very little to bring it "to taste."

I sincerely hope you find learning all the wonderful alternative ways that you can season a dish as fun and exciting as I have. Sharing that knowledge with you in this book has been a joy as well. Enjoy and dine in good health!

Pamela Rice Hahn

The EVERYTHING® Series

Editorial

Publishing Director	Gary M. Krebs
Managing Editor	Kate McBride
Copy Chief	Laura MacLaughlin
Acquisitions Editor	Bethany Brown
Development Editor	Karen Johnson Jacot
Production Editor	Jamie Wielgus

Production

Production Director	Susan Beale
Production Manager	Michelle Roy Kelly
Series Designers	Daria Perreault
	Colleen Cunningham
Cover Design	Paul Beatrice
	Frank Rivera
Layout and Graphics	Colleen Cunningham
	Rachael Eiben
	Michelle Roy Kelly
	John Paulhus
	Daria Perreault
	Erin Ring
Series Cover Artist	Barry Littmann

THE
EVERYTHING®
LOW-SALT
COOKBOOK

300 flavorful recipes to help reduce your sodium intake

Pamela Rice Hahn

Adams Media
Avon, Massachusetts

To all my visitors at CookingWithPam.com

An Everything® Series Book.
Everything® and everything.com® are registered trademarks of F+W Media, Inc.
Published by Adams Media, a division of F+W Media, Inc.
57 Littlefield Street, Avon, MA 02322 U.S.A.
www.adamsmedia.com
ISBN 10: 1-59337-044-X
ISBN 13: 978-1-59337-044-2
Printed in the United States of America.

J I H G F E D

Library of Congress Cataloging-in-Publication Data
Hahn, Pamela Rice.
The everything low-salt cookbook / Pamela Rice Hahn.
p.   cm.
ISBN 1-59337-044-X
1. Salt-free diet–Recipes. I. Title. II. Series: Everything series.
RM237.8.H346 2004
641.5'6323–dc22

2003023147

This publication is designed to provide accurate and authoritative information with regard to the subject matter covered. It is sold with the understanding that the publisher is not engaged in rendering legal, accounting, or other professional advice. If legal advice or other expert assistance is required, the services of a competent professional person should be sought.
    —From a *Declaration of Principles* jointly adopted by a Committee of the American Bar Association and a Committee of Publishers and Associations

Many of the designations used by manufacturers and sellers to distinguish their products are claimed as trademarks. Where those designations appear in this book and Adams Media was aware of a trademark claim, the designations have been printed with initial capital letters.

The Everything® *Low-Salt Cookbook* is intended as a reference volume only, not as a medical manual. In light of the complex, individual, and specific nature of health problems, this book is not intended to replace professional medical advice. The ideas, procedures, and suggestions in this book are intended to supplement, not replace, the advice of a trained medical professional. Consult your physician before adopting the suggestions in this book, as well as about any condition that may require diagnosis or medical attention. The author and publisher disclaim any liability arising directly or indirectly from the use of this book.

This book is available at quantity discounts for bulk purchases.
For information, call 1-800-289-0963.

Contents

Acknowledgments

For their help and support, I would like to thank everyone at Adams Media. For all of their hard work and perseverance, I would like to thank my agent Sheree Bykofsky and her associates Janet Rosen and Megan Buckley. Special thanks also goes to my daughter Lara Sutton and the other joys in my life: Taylor, Charlie, and Courtney; Andrew, Tony, Dennis, and Ann Rice; my mother and sister Tam; my niece Nicole; my photographer buddy who makes house calls, Bill Grunden; my computer guru Don Lachey; Doris Meinerding, the most helpful and friendliest Realtor in the world; and David Hebert, Eric J. Ehlers, Jodi Cornelius, and my other online friends.

Introduction

▶ SALT IS AN ESSENTIAL PART OF OUR DIETS. In fact, human blood is 0.9 percent sodium chloride (salt). That salt in the blood helps maintain the electrolyte balance inside and outside of cells. While individual needs can vary, most studies indicate that the human body needs only around 500 milligrams of salt a day to maintain that healthy balance—but that 500 milligrams is a fraction of what many Americans consume in a day. So much salt is present in processed foods that consuming 1,200 to 2,000 milligrams is now often considered a salt-restricted diet. The average American consumes 3,300 milligrams a day. The American Heart Association recommends a maximum of 2,400 milligrams a day.

To give you an idea of how much salt constitutes the recommended target milligrams a day, consider these "straight from the salt shaker" statistics:

- ¼ teaspoon salt = 500 milligrams sodium
- ½ teaspoon salt = 1,000 milligrams sodium
- ¾ teaspoon salt = 1,500 milligrams sodium
- 1 teaspoon salt = 2,000 milligrams sodium
- 1 teaspoon baking soda = 1,000 milligrams sodium

The Benefits of Less Salt

Most people are aware that too much salt in the diet can cause an increase in blood pressure in salt-sensitive individuals. An elevation in blood pressure increases the risk of stroke. In addition to blood pressure and the risk of cardiac health concerns, too much sodium can cause other problems as well. For example, a study reported in the May 1996 issue of *American Journal of Clinical Nutrition* found that excess salt in the diet can increase calcium loss, which in turn exacerbates the risk of osteoporosis. Excess salt in the diet has been shown to increase the risk of stomach cancer, ulcers, and migraines. To complicate matters even more, some salt-sensitive individuals exhibit normal blood pressure levels yet retain salt in the kidneys instead of excreting it in their urine. Thus, salt sensitivity alone (without the telltale warning signs of high blood pressure or fluid retention) can still increase the risk of death.

Chances are that reducing the salt in your diet won't be the only lifestyle change suggestion your doctor or dietician makes, but, for some, it can be the most intimidating one. Increasing the amount of daily exercise can be as simple as climbing some stairs instead of taking the elevator or parking the car a little further from your destination and walking the additional distance.

Cutting Back

Once you start looking for ways to cut down on the salt in your diet, you realize that salt is seemingly everywhere! Even when it isn't listed as a named ingredient on a food label, it can be present in many food preservatives. It's in the baking soda used to leaven baked goods. A fast-food chicken sandwich isn't normally thought of as a "salty food," yet it can contain more than 1,100 milligrams of sodium. A serving of canned soup can contain almost that much! Because of today's fast-paced lifestyle, you, too, probably rely to a certain extent on fast foods–whether you get them at a drive-up window or in the form of a convenience food at the supermarket.

Therefore, the task of cutting back on salt is already complicated for those who only want to reduce sodium consumption to the 2,400 milligrams a day recommended by the American Heart Association. If you have already developed a health concern that requires that you consume a reduced-salt diet, you'll need to pay even closer attention to food labels from now on. Regardless of which category you currently fall in, you can probably now better understand why it's important to control your sodium consumption.

Today's refined table salt is a single chemical compound, sodium chloride. Not only is table salt stripped of more than sixty trace minerals and essential macronutrients, it's then bleached and anticaking agents are added so it's easier to pour or sprinkle. This results in a chemical that's difficult for the body to absorb and digest, which then causes the health problems mentioned earlier, such as high blood pressure.

For that reason, many people find that their body is better able to handle the salt they ingest if that salt is in a form closest to its natural state as possible. Sodium content will be the same whether you're using table salt or sea salt, but you may find that because of its purer, less chemical flavor, it takes less sea salt to season food. Kosher salt can also be an alternative but, because of its larger crystals, it doesn't always absorb as well—and for some people it takes more kosher salt than table or sea salt to achieve the desired effect. For that reason, as far as the recipes in this book are concerned, table salt or sea salt are interchangeable. Unless your dietician provides you with specific instructions to the contrary, it's your choice as to whether you use table or sea salt.

In addition to cutting down on how much salt you add to your food, making wise choices about which ingredients you use when preparing meals can make a big difference. While there are now other reduced-sodium (and reduced- or no-fat) products on the market, the nutritional analyses for those products vary widely. Reduced-sodium foods often contain more sugar; reduced-fat foods usually contain more sodium than do regular products.

When choosing a shortcut, always try to pick the one that offers the lowest sodium content. To help you recognize what those labels mean when you're looking for low-sodium products, here are the common explanations for what the phrases on those labels mean:

- **Sodium-Free**: 5 milligrams or less of sodium per serving
- **Very Low Sodium:** 35 milligrams or less of sodium per serving
- **Low Sodium:** 140 milligrams or less of sodium per serving
- **Reduced or Less Sodium:** A minimum of 25 percent less sodium than the regular version
- **Light in Sodium:** 50 percent less sodium than the regular version
- **Salt-Free:** 5 milligrams or less of sodium per serving
- **Low Sodium Meal:** 140 milligrams or less of sodium per 100 grams
- **No Added Salt or Unsalted:** a product that no salt was added to during processing; however, this does not mean that the product does not contain sodium, as there can be sodium occurring naturally in the food

Understanding Nutritional Analyses in This Book

Unless stated otherwise, some foods—like cottage cheese, for example—are factored into the nutritional analysis using a generic average. Other times named products are used and the nutritional analysis was done using that specific product. The sodium content of products is all over the map, so be very careful about making substitutions.

When a choice is given between two ingredients in a recipe in this book, the nutritional analysis was done using the first ingredient. Oftentimes, the ingredient will be one from a recipe in this book. In that instance, the nutritional analysis information for the portion used is what was used to calculate the entire recipe. Therefore, if you plan to substitute a commercial ingredient, consult that ingredient's recipe for the nutritional analysis so that you can make an accurate comparison, and adjust the recipe accordingly, if necessary. The same thing applies to named ingredients. For example, Hellmann's or Best Foods mayonnaise is a named brand mentioned in several recipes. That doesn't mean you can't substitute another brand; however, you should consult the sodium content for the brand you have on hand or wish to use as the substitute to ensure that it isn't higher in sodium than the ingredient suggested in a recipe.

When a recipe calls for a food prepared from another recipe in this book, the nutritional analysis *includes* that food in the counts.

NutriBase IV Clinical program was used to calculate the nutritional analysis for the recipes in this book. Named brand products are used when it's essential to do so to give an accurate reading of the nutritional analysis for the recipe. As already stated, that doesn't mean you can't substitute other similar ingredients. It does, however, mean that you need to be careful about checking the package to make sure you're not adding something that's higher in sodium.

Low-Salt Cooking Tips

Keep in mind that you can use a seasoning blend even when a recipe in this book mentions individual seasonings. Simply substitute the blend that has similar seasonings.

Additional essentials for your pantry should include dried lemon granules, 100% lemon juice (not the bottled kind made from concentrate, but like that found in the freezer case from Minute Maid), dried minced onion and garlic, good-quality onion and garlic powders, nonfat dry milk, and no-salt-added instant mashed potatoes. While they're not mandatory, stocking some freeze-dried ingredients like shallots and minced green onion (scallion) are great to have on hand, too, because of their almost instantaneous ability to reconstitute in a dish.

Likewise, while many cooking experts suggest replacing spices and herbs every six months to a year, that isn't because spices stored properly in a cool, dry place go stale. Rather, even when they're stored properly, the intensity of those spices and herbs do diminish over time. That decrease in flavor isn't the end of the world, however; in most cases, you can simply use more.

Specific information about products used in this book is mentioned in Appendix B, such as which type of "large, deep nonstick sauté pan" was used to test the recipes. That reference, listed often in the book, refers to a 3½-quart oven-safe skillet, which is large enough for most of the recipes in the book and can also be used on the stovetop and then moved to the oven to finish off a dish, when necessary.

You'll also notice that the suggestion is made to treat even nonstick cookware with nonstick cooking spray. That's because over time small scratches can form on the nonstick surface, which can cause food to stick. Another benefit is that when you first use a nonstick spray, it takes far less oil to sauté vegetables.

There's also another "lower-fat frying" *and* lower-sodium benefit possible when you first treat a nonstick pan with nonstick spray or spray oil. For those times when only some fried meat will satisfy your craving, you'll use far less oil if you rinse the meat in cold water and then dry it between paper towels, rub a little oil over the surface of the meat, and then use a salt-free seasoning blend on both sides of the meat. Bring the nonstick pan to temperature and then fry the meat as usual. Such instructions normally suggest salting the surface of the meat before it's fried, because the salt helps draw the extra moisture to the surface of the meat so that it evaporates quickly. This causes the meat to sear, which is essential for that caramelized "fried" taste. But drying the meat between the paper towels eliminates the need to use salt to draw the moisture to the surface because you've already removed that moisture with towels!

The most important thing to keep in mind as you experiment with new seasoning sensations while you adapt to your new low-salt eating lifestyle is that you're making a commitment to better manage your health. Making, and sticking with, that commitment to eat a healthy diet literally can be your life or death decision.

CHAPTER 1
Appetizers and Finger Foods

Steamer Clams in Ginger Sauce

Serves 28	
Per serving:	
Calories:	10.19
Protein:	1.65 g
Carbohydrates:	0.81 g
Total fat:	0.02 g
Sat. fat:	0.00 g
Cholesterol:	2.50 mg
Sodium:	88.51 mg
Fiber:	0.33 g

2 teaspoons Bragg Liquid Aminos
1 teaspoon lemon juice
¼ cup spring onions, thinly sliced
1 teaspoon white rice wine
  vinegar
4 teaspoons apple juice
1 teaspoon ground ginger
¼ teaspoon Oriental mustard
  powder

4 cloves garlic, minced, or
  1 teaspoon garlic powder
1 teaspoon dried green onion
  flakes
¼ teaspoon granulated sugar
1 (15-ounce) Gordon's Chesapeake
  Classics Cocktail Clams (Steamer
  Size), drained
1 large cucumber

1. In a bowl, combine all ingredients except the steamer clams and cucumber. Add the drained clams and toss to mix.
2. Wash and slice the cucumber. Arrange the cucumber slices on a platter and place a clam atop each slice. Chill until ready to serve.

Onion Dip

Serves 16	
Per serving:	
Calories:	33.51
Protein:	1.01 g
Carbohydrates:	1.21 g
Total fat:	2.79 g
Sat. fat:	1.61 g
Cholesterol:	8.19 mg
Sodium:	33.54 mg
Fiber:	0.02 g

2 teaspoons onion powder
½ teaspoon dried green onion
  flakes
⅛ teaspoon dried granulated
  roasted garlic
⅛ teaspoon dried or freeze-dried
  chopped chives
⅛ teaspoon dried parsley
⅛ teaspoon celery seed

⅛ teaspoon dry mustard
½ cup plain nonfat yogurt
4 ounces cream cheese, at room
  temperature
1 tablespoon Hellmann's or Best
  Foods Real Mayonnaise
1 teaspoon Lea & Perrins
  Worcestershire sauce

Add all ingredients to a small bowl and mix to combine. Cover and refrigerate until needed.

Sweet Stuff Guacamole Dip

1 avocado
1½ teaspoons apple cider vinegar
1 clove garlic
1 teaspoon Bragg Liquid Aminos
½ teaspoon Lea & Perrins
   Worcestershire sauce

2 teaspoons extra-virgin olive oil
2 tablespoons apple juice
½ cup plain nonfat yogurt
1 teaspoon fresh lemon juice

Put all ingredients in a food processor or blender and process until smooth. Serve with unsalted tortilla chips.

Serves 16	
Per serving:	
Calories:	31.50
Protein:	0.76 g
Carbohydrates:	2.12 g
Total fat:	2.44 g
Sat. fat:	0.39 g
Cholesterol:	0.39 mg
Sodium:	29.56 mg
Fiber:	0.64 g

Garlic Toast

Spectrum Naturals Extra Virgin
   Olive Spray Oil
4 (1-ounce) slices French Bread
   (page 216)

1 clove garlic, cut in half lengthwise

1. Preheat oven to 350°.
2. Using the spray oil (or an oil mister filled with extra-virgin olive oil), lightly spray both sides of each slice of bread. Arrange the bread slices on a baking sheet. Bake for 6 to 8 minutes.
3. Remove from oven. Handle the toasted bread slices carefully so that you don't burn your fingers, and rub the cut side of the garlic clove across the top of each slice. Serve warm.

Serves 4	
Per serving:	
Calories:	77.06
Protein:	2.31 g
Carbohydrates:	16.06 g
Total fat:	0.22 g
Sat. fat:	0.03 g
Cholesterol:	0.00 mg
Sodium:	24.85 mg
Fiber:	0.65 g

Open-Face Wild Mushroom Wontons

Serves 24	
Per serving:	
Calories:	54.23
Protein:	2.50 g
Carbohydrates:	6.72 g
Total fat:	2.06 g
Sat. fat:	0.92 g
Cholesterol:	5.12 mg
Sodium:	72.42 mg
Fiber:	0.50 g

1 tablespoon olive or canola oil
1 tablespoon unsalted butter
½ cup sliced shallots
½ teaspoon freshly ground black pepper
¾ pound assorted wild mushrooms (such as chanterelle, wood ear, shiitake, morel), cleaned, stemmed, and thinly sliced
¾ cup water
¾ teaspoon Minor's Low Sodium Chicken Base
¼ cup instant nonfat dry milk
½ cup ricotta cheese
½ teaspoon herbal seasoning blend of your choice
24 wonton wrappers
Spectrum Naturals Extra Virgin Olive Spray Oil
2 tablespoons grated Parmesan cheese

1. Preheat oven to 375°.
2. In a large, heavy nonstick skillet, heat the oil and melt the butter over medium-high heat. Add the shallots and cook, stirring, for 1 minute. Add the pepper and mushrooms; sauté until the mushrooms become soft and most of the mushroom liquid is evaporated, about 8 minutes.
3. Add the water and heat until it begins to boil. Dissolve the Minor's base in the water. Reduce heat and add the nonfat dry milk, whisking to combine with the mushroom mixture. Add the ricotta cheese and herbal seasoning, and mix to combine; cook until heated through. Remove from heat.
4. Line a baking sheet with nonstick aluminum foil. Prepare the wonton wrappers by lightly spraying one side of each with the spray oil. Place sprayed-side down on the foil. Evenly divide the mushroom mixture, placing a spoonful on each wonton wrapper. Top the mushroom mixture with the grated cheese.
5. Bake for 8 to 10 minutes or until the wontons are brown and crunchy and the cheese is melted and bubbly.

Herbed Provence-Style Flatbread (Fougasse)

Basic White Bread dough (page 212)
2 tablespoons extra-virgin olive oil
½ teaspoon dried rosemary
¼ teaspoon dried French thyme
¼ teaspoon dried tarragon
¼ teaspoon dried basil
¼ teaspoon dried savory
¼ teaspoon dried fennel seeds

¼ teaspoon dried lavender
⅛ teaspoon dried marjoram
⅛ teaspoon freshly ground black pepper
2 tablespoons grated Parmesan cheese
Spectrum Naturals Extra Virgin Olive Spray Oil

Serves 24	
Per serving:	
Calories:	98.79
Protein:	2.39 g
Carbohydrates:	16.15 g
Total fat:	2.59 g
Sat. fat:	0.42 g
Cholesterol:	0.33 mg
Sodium:	105.16 mg
Fiber:	0.60 g

1. Preheat oven to 450°.
2. Remove the prepared basic bread dough from the refrigerator and punch it down. Lightly coat your hands with olive oil. Divide the dough into 24 equal pieces, shaping each piece into a ball. Set aside to rest for a few minutes.
3. Mix together the rosemary, thyme, tarragon, basil, savory, fennel seeds, lavender, marjoram, and pepper. Use a mortar and pestle or spice grinder to process into a coarse meal. Stir in the Parmesan cheese.
4. Using your hands, flatten each ball of dough. (Flatten into irregular shapes to give character to the bread.) Spray a baking sheet with the olive oil spray and place the dough on the sheet. With a pastry scraper, *lame* (a tool used to slit the tops of bread loaves), or X-acto knife (kept specifically for that purpose), cut 3 or 4 lengthwise slashes into the bread. Gently pull apart at the slashes. Cover with a clean towel, and let rest for 10 minutes.
5. Brush lightly with olive oil, then sprinkle with the herb-Parmesan cheese topping. Bake until golden and crusty, about 15 to 18 minutes.

❀ When Using a Bread Stone . . .

If baking Fougasse on a bread stone, skip using the olive oil spray and dust your bread and the stone with cornmeal to prevent the flatbreads from sticking.

Shrimp Toasts

Serves 48	
Per serving:	
Calories:	42.35
Protein:	2.92 g
Carbohydrates:	4.50 g
Total fat:	1.33 g
Sat. fat:	0.60 g
Cholesterol:	17.02 mg
Sodium:	49.03 mg
Fiber:	0.17 g

1 pound peeled shrimp
¼ cup minced green onions
2 tablespoons minced fresh cilantro
1 teaspoon minced garlic
1 teaspoon minced jalapeño pepper
1 large egg white
1 tablespoon nonfat dry milk
4 ounces cream cheese, cut into pieces

½ cup plain nonfat yogurt
12 (1-ounce) slices Basic White Bread (page 212), crusts removed
Spectrum Naturals Extra Virgin Olive Spray Oil with Garlic Flavor
Spectrum Naturals Canola Spray Oil with Butter Flavor

1. Preheat the oven to 375°.
2. In a food processor, combine the shrimp, green onions, cilantro, garlic, jalapeño, egg white, and nonfat dry milk; process until smooth. Add cubes of cream cheese and pulse to incorporate. Add the yogurt and pulse just until incorporated, being careful not to overprocess.
3. To shorten the baking time and help ensure that the bread is crisp in the center, first toast it; then spray the bottom of each slice of bread with a light amount of the garlic-flavored spray oil. Evenly divide the shrimp mixture between the slices of bread, spreading it on the nonsprayed side of the bread and making sure to spread it to the edges of the bread.
4. Place the coated bread slices (shrimp mixture side up) on a baking sheet treated with nonstick spray or covered with nonstick foil. Lightly spray the tops of the bread with the butter-flavored spray oil. Bake for 10 to 15 minutes, or until the bread is crisp and the shrimp topping bubbles and is lightly browned. Use a pizza cutter or serrated knife to cut each slice of bread into 4 equal pieces. Arrange on a tray or platter and serve immediately.

❈ Saving Some Steps
There's no reason to take the time to remove the crusts from home-made bread slice by slice. Before you slice the bread, cut off the crusts. Then slice the bread into 1-ounce pieces.

Baked Savory Lemon-Pepper Cheesecake

20 Health Valley Low Fat Sesame Crackers
8 ounces cream cheese, softened
16 ounces nonfat cottage cheese
4 large eggs
1 tablespoon unbleached all-purpose flour
½ cup skim milk
1 cup shredded Swiss cheese
¼ cup grated Parmesan cheese
2 green onions, chopped
1 teaspoon lemon zest
½ teaspoon freshly ground black pepper
Optional: Pinch of dried red pepper flakes or cayenne pepper
Optional: Assorted crackers and raw vegetable strips

Serves 16	
Per serving:	
Calories:	149.97
Protein:	11.33 g
Carbohydrates:	4.70 g
Total fat:	9.44 g
Sat. fat:	5.35 g
Cholesterol:	79.67 mg
Sodium:	151.02 mg
Fiber:	0.29 g

1. Preheat oven to 350°.
2. Prepare the "crust" by crushing the crackers—either by placing them in a plastic bag and rolling a rolling pin over them or by putting them through a food processor or blender. Spread evenly in a 9" spring-form pan.
3. Add the cream cheese, cottage cheese, eggs, flour, and milk to the bowl of a food processor. (A few cracker crumbs remaining in the bowl won't alter the recipe, but if they bother you, wipe out the bowl first.) Process until smooth. Add the Swiss cheese, Parmesan cheese, onions, lemon peel, pepper, and red pepper (or cayenne), if using. Process until blended.
4. Carefully spoon the cheese mixture over the crackers in the springform pan. Bake for 1 hour or until the top is light golden brown. (The mixture may not be firmed up in the center; it will get firm as it cools.)
5. Set the pan on a wire rack to cool the cheesecake to room temperature. Cover and refrigerate for at least 4 hours or overnight before serving. Serve with crackers and raw vegetables.

❋ Softening Cream Cheese
Place completely unwrapped package of cream cheese on microwave-safe plate. Microwave on high for 15 seconds. Turn the plate and microwave on high for 5-second increments until slightly softened.

Roasted Garlic and Red Pepper Hummus

Serves 32	
(1 tbsp per serving)	
Per serving:	
Calories:	32.57
Protein:	1.39 g
Carbohydrates:	3.89 g
Total fat:	1.47 g
Sat. fat:	0.20 g
Cholesterol:	0.00 mg
Sodium:	2.67 mg
Fiber:	1.05 g

2 cloves Roasted Garlic (page 248)
2 cups cooked (no salt added)
  garbanzo beans, drained
⅓ cup tahini
⅓ cup lemon juice

½ cup chopped roasted red peppers (see instructions for roasting peppers on page 58)
¼ teaspoon dried basil
Freshly ground black pepper

In a food processor, combine the garlic, garbanzo beans, tahini, lemon juice, chopped red peppers, and basil. Process until the mixture is smooth. Season to taste with freshly ground pepper. Transfer the hummus to a covered bowl and chill until ready to serve.

Easy Bread "Sticks"

Serves 4	
Per serving:	
Calories:	77.06
Protein:	2.31 g
Carbohydrates:	16.06 g
Total fat:	0.22 g
Sat. fat:	0.03 g
Cholesterol:	0.00 mg
Sodium:	24.85 mg
Fiber:	0.65 g

4 (1-ounce) thinly sliced French
  Bread (page 216) crusts

Olive oil

1. Preheat over to 350°.
2. Using an oil mister, lightly spray both sides of each slice of bread with olive oil. Arrange on a baking sheet.
3. Bake for 5 to 10 minutes. (Baking time will depend on the size and thickness of the crusts and on how crisp you want the bread "sticks.")

Sweet Pea Guacamole

3 tablespoons extra-virgin olive oil
2 tablespoons fresh lime juice
2 tablespoons minced fresh
   coriander
2 jalapeño peppers, seeded and
   minced
½ teaspoon ground cumin
½ teaspoon ground coriander
½ teaspoon ground black pepper

1 (16-ounce) package Cascadian
   Farm Organic frozen Garden
   Peas, cooked without salt and
   drained
2 plum tomatoes, peeled, seeded,
   and diced
1 small red onion, finely diced
Optional: Honey or jalapeño jelly,
   to taste

Serves 8	
Per serving:	
Calories:	102.38
Protein:	3.11 g
Carbohydrates:	10.48 g
Total fat:	5.15 g
Sat. fat:	0.69 g
Cholesterol:	0.00 mg
Sodium:	66.78 mg
Fiber:	3.20 g

1. In the bowl of a food processor, combine the oil, lime juice,
   coriander leaves, peppers, spices, and black pepper; process until
   smooth.
2. Add the peas. Pulse a few times to chop the peas and combine with
   the other ingredients.
3. Use a spatula to scrape the mixture into a serving bowl. Stir in the
   tomatoes and onion. Check seasoning and adjust if necessary, adding
   some honey or jalapeño jelly if a touch of sweetness is necessary to
   mellow the hotness of the peppers.

❀ Hidden Sodium

*Frozen peas are sorted by size in saltwater baths. As a result, they'll
already have a higher sodium content than fresh ones. If you use
frozen peas, make sure you use a "no additional salt added" variety.
Using the "worst-case scenario" formula, the nutritional analysis for
the Sweet Pea Guacamole recipe was calculated using the named
brand frozen peas that have 95 milligrams of sodium per ⅔ cup
serving; other brands may vary.*

Tomato Butter Toasts

Serves 48	
Per serving:	
Calories:	41.42
Protein:	1.32 g
Carbohydrates:	4.63 g
Total fat:	1.90 g
Sat. fat:	1.06 g
Cholesterol:	4.23 mg
Sodium:	62.24 mg
Fiber:	0.21 g

¾ cup Tomato Butter (page 249)
¼ cup minced green onions
2 tablespoons minced fresh basil
4 cloves garlic, minced
12 (1-ounce) slices Basic White
  Bread (page 212), crusts removed
Spectrum Naturals Extra Virgin Olive
  Spray Oil with Garlic Flavor
¾ cup grated Parmesan cheese

1. Preheat oven to 375°.
2. In the bowl of a food processor, combine the tomato butter, green onions, basil, and garlic; process until mixed.
3. To shorten the baking time and help ensure that the bread is crisp in the center, first toast it. Spray the bottom of each slice of bread with a light amount of the garlic-flavored spray oil. Evenly divide the tomato-butter mixture between the slices of bread, spreading it on the nonsprayed side of the bread and making sure to spread it to the edges of the bread. Evenly sprinkle 1 tablespoon of the Parmesan cheese over the top of each piece of coated bread.
4. Place the coated bread slices (tomato-butter mixture side up) on a baking sheet treated with nonstick spray or covered with nonstick foil. Bake for 10 to 12 minutes or until the bread is crisp and the topping bubbles and is lightly browned. Use a pizza cutter or serrated knife to cut each slice of bread into 4 equal pieces. Arrange on a tray or platter and serve immediately.

❁ Peeling Tomatoes

To peel a tomato, first cut out the stem and then slice a shallow X on the bottom end of the tomato. Plunge the tomato into boiling water for a few seconds, and then remove with a slotted spoon. Immediately plunge the tomato into ice water (to stop the cooking process and loosen the skin). Once the tomato is cooled, remove it from the ice water and use a paring knife to peel away the skin.

Honey-Spiced Almonds

2 tablespoons unsalted butter
½ teaspoon cinnamon
⅛ teaspoon ground cloves
⅛ teaspoon ground ginger

½ cup honey
½ teaspoon orange zest
3 cups raw almonds

Serves 12	
Per serving:	
Calories:	98.59
Protein:	2.56 g
Carbohydrates:	8.16 g
Total fat:	6.97 g
Sat. fat:	1.06 g
Cholesterol:	2.59 mg
Sodium:	0.53 mg
Fiber:	1.42 g

1. Put the butter, spices, honey, and orange zest in a large microwave-safe bowl. Microwave on high for 1 minute or until the butter is melted. Stir well to combine.
2. Add the almonds to the honey mixture and stir well to combine. Microwave on high for 3 minutes; stir well. Microwave on high for another 3 minutes; stir. Spread the nuts on a nonstick foil-lined baking sheet to cool. Be careful—the mixture will be very hot!

Honey-Almond Spread

2 tablespoons fresh orange juice
½ cup chopped raisins
1 tablespoon honey
4 ounces cream cheese

½ cup plain nonfat yogurt
¼ cup chopped Honey-Spiced
   Almonds

Serves 32 (1 tablespoon each)	
Per serving:	
Calories:	26.65
Protein:	0.63 g
Carbohydrates:	3.05 g
Total fat:	1.47 g
Sat. fat:	0.82 g
Cholesterol:	4.05 mg
Sodium:	13.53 mg
Fiber:	0.14 g

1. Mix together the orange juice and raisins; set aside.
2. In a small bowl, mix together the honey, cream cheese, and yogurt. Stir the chopped raisins-orange juice mixture and almonds into the cream cheese mixture. Cover, and chill in the refrigerator until ready to serve.

Pissaladiere (Onion Tart)

Serves 24	
Per serving:	
Calories:	55.76
Protein:	1.46 g
Carbohydrates:	9.33 g
Total fat:	1.38 g
Sat. fat:	0.25 g
Cholesterol:	0.33 mg
Sodium:	56.86 mg
Fiber:	0.46 g

¼ teaspoon dried lemon granules, crushed
¼ teaspoon mustard powder
1 tablespoon water
1 tablespoon extra-virgin olive oil
2 large sweet onions, thinly sliced
4 medium-sized cloves garlic, finely chopped
1 fresh bay leaf
¼ teaspoon dried thyme, crushed
2 teaspoons dried parsley, crushed
¼ teaspoon freshly ground black pepper
Pinch dried red pepper flakes
½ recipe Basic White Bread dough (page 212)
2 tablespoons grated Parmesan cheese

1. Preheat oven to 450° with a rack set in the center position.
2. Add the lemon granules and mustard powder to a small microwave-safe bowl or coffee cup; spoon the water and oil over the top. Microwave on high for 30 seconds; cover with plastic wrap and set aside.
3. Add the onions, garlic, and bay leaf to a microwave-safe bowl. Cover and microwave on high for 4 minutes. Turn the bowl and microwave on high for an additional 3 minutes. (Be careful not to burn the onions.) Carefully remove the cover (there will be lots of steam!). Discard the bay leaf and mix in the thyme, parsley, pepper, and red pepper flakes; cover and set aside.
4. Treat a 13" × 18" rimmed baking sheet (jelly roll pan) with spray oil. Place the dough on a lightly floured surface and roll the dough into a 13" × 18" rectangle; transfer to the baking pan. Cover with a damp cotton towel or plastic wrap and let rest for 30 minutes to rise. (The dough may "shrink" away from the edges of pan; if so, gently use the tips of your fingers to push it back to the edges.) Prick the dough all over with the tines of a fork. Uncover the lemon granules mixture and whisk with a fork. Brush the mixture evenly over the dough.
5. Stir the Parmesan cheese into the cooked onion mixture; spread the mixture evenly over the prepared dough. Bake for 12 minutes. Rotate the pan; bake until the crust is cooked through and the edges are lightly browned, about 12 minutes more. Remove from oven and transfer the tart to a serving board. Slice and serve warm or at room temperature.

Carbonara Tart

¾ teaspoon Minor's Bacon Base

1 tablespoon water

1 tablespoon extra-virgin olive oil

2 large sweet onions, thinly sliced

4 medium-sized cloves garlic, finely chopped

1 fresh bay leaf

¼ teaspoon dried thyme, crushed

2 teaspoons dried parsley, crushed

¼ teaspoon freshly ground black pepper

Pinch dried red pepper flakes

½ recipe Basic White Bread dough (page 212)

4 eggs, beaten

2 tablespoons grated Parmesan cheese

Serves 24	
Per serving:	
Calories:	68.84
Protein:	2.52 g
Carbohydrates:	9.47 g
Total fat:	2.27 g
Sat. fat:	0.53 g
Cholesterol:	35.80 mg
Sodium:	95.61 mg
Fiber:	0.46 g

1. Preheat oven to 450° with a rack set in the center position.
2. Add the bacon base to a small microwave-safe bowl or coffee cup; spoon the water and oil over the top. Microwave on high for 30 seconds; cover with plastic wrap and set aside.
3. Add the onions, garlic, and bay leaf to a microwave-safe bowl. Cover and microwave on high for 4 minutes. Turn the bowl and microwave on high for an additional 3 minutes. (Be careful not to burn the onions.) Carefully remove the cover (there will be lots of steam!); discard the bay leaf and mix in the thyme, parsley, pepper, and red pepper flakes; cover and set aside to cool.
4. Treat a 13" × 18" rimmed baking sheet (jelly roll pan) with spray oil. Place the dough on a lightly floured surface and roll the dough into a 13" × 18" rectangle; transfer to the baking pan. Cover with a damp cotton towel or plastic wrap and let rest for 30 minutes to rise. (The dough may "shrink" away from edges of pan; if so, gently use the tips of your fingers to push it back to the edges.) Prick the dough all over with the tines of a fork. Uncover the bacon base mixture and whisk with a fork. Brush the mixture evenly over the dough.
5. Stir the eggs and Parmesan cheese into the cooked onion mixture; spread the mixture evenly over the prepared dough. Bake for 12 minutes. Rotate the pan and bake until the crust is cooked through and the edges are lightly browned, about 12 minutes more. Remove from oven and transfer the tart to a serving board. Slice and serve warm or at room temperature.

Greek Onion Tart

Serves 24	
Per serving:	
Calories:	64.48
Protein:	1.45 g
Carbohydrates:	9.37 g
Total fat:	2.26 g
Sat. fat:	0.35 g
Cholesterol:	1.05 mg
Sodium:	177.29 mg
Fiber:	0.46 g

¼ *teaspoon dried lemon granules, crushed*
¼ *teaspoon mustard powder*
1 *tablespoon water*
1 *tablespoon extra-virgin olive oil*
2 *large sweet onions, thinly sliced*
4 *medium-sized cloves garlic, finely chopped*
1 *fresh bay leaf*

¼ *teaspoon dried thyme, crushed*
2 *teaspoons dried parsley, crushed*
¼ *teaspoon freshly ground black pepper*
Pinch dried red pepper flakes
½ *recipe Basic White Bread dough (page 212)*
12 *pitted calamata olives, sliced*
1 *ounce feta cheese, crumbled*

1. Preheat oven to 450° with a rack set in the center position.
2. Add the lemon granules and mustard powder to a small microwave-safe bowl or coffee cup; spoon the water and oil over the top. Microwave on high for 30 seconds; cover with plastic wrap and set aside.
3. Add the onions, garlic, and bay leaf to a microwave-safe bowl; microwave, covered, on high for 4 minutes. Turn the bowl and microwave on high for an additional 3 minutes. Carefully remove the cover; discard the bay leaf and mix in the thyme, parsley, pepper, and red pepper flakes; cover and set aside.
4. Treat a 13" × 18" rimmed baking sheet (jelly roll pan) with spray oil. Place the dough on a lightly floured surface and roll dough into a 13" × 18" rectangle; transfer the dough to the baking pan. Cover with a damp cotton towel or plastic wrap and let rest for 30 minutes to rise. (The dough may "shrink" away from the edges of the pan; if so, gently use the tips of your fingers to push it back to the edges.) Prick the dough all over with the tines of a fork. Uncover the lemon granules mixture and whisk with a fork. Brush the mixture evenly over the dough.
5. Stir the olives into the cooked onion mixture; spread the mixture evenly over the prepared dough. Sprinkle the feta cheese over the top of the onions. Bake for 12 minutes. Rotate the pan and bake until the crust is cooked through and the edges are lightly browned, about 12 minutes more. Remove from oven; slice and serve warm or at room temperature.

Chicken Salad Mold

½ cup plain nonfat yogurt

2 envelopes unflavored gelatin

1¼ cups water

¾ teaspoon Minor's Low Sodium Chicken Base

¼ teaspoon Minor's Roasted Mirepoix Flavor Concentrate

¼ cup Maple Leaf Potato Granules

1 teaspoon cider vinegar

1 tablespoon lemon juice

1 teaspoon Dijon mustard

1 teaspoon brown sugar

1 tablespoon Hellmann's or Best Foods Real Mayonnaise

½ cup nonfat cottage cheese

4 ounces cream cheese

1 teaspoon celery seeds

1 teaspoon dried celery flakes

½ cup Cascadian Farm Dill Relish

¼ cup chopped green onion (scallions)

¼ teaspoon mustard powder

⅛ teaspoon freshly ground pepper

1 teaspoon Country Table Spice Blend (page 275)

1½ pounds cooked, chopped chicken

Serves 24	
Per serving:	
Calories:	108.59
Protein:	10.95 g
Carbohydrates:	3.36 g
Total fat:	5.63 g
Sat. fat:	1.99 g
Cholesterol:	29.23 mg
Sodium:	261.40 mg
Fiber:	0.49 g

1. Add the yogurt to a blender or food processor and sprinkle the gelatin on top; let stand for 2 minutes to soften the gelatin. Bring the water to a boil, then add the boiling water to the yogurt mixture and process until the gelatin dissolves. Add the remaining ingredients *except* for the chicken and process until smooth. Fold in the chopped chicken.
2. Taste for seasonings. You can add herbs like chopped chives, a little more cider vinegar, or some freshly ground black pepper without affecting the sodium content. Pour into a mold or terrine treated with nonstick spray and chill in the refrigerator until firm.

❃ Even Less Sodium . . .

The nutritional analysis for the Chicken Salad Mold recipe was done using the "worst-case scenario" of assuming that the chicken was prepared in a manner similar to the suggestions in the Easy Slow-Cooked Chicken recipe (page 151). The mold will have a lower sodium content if you use unseasoned, cooked light- and dark-meat chicken.

Italian-Style Baked Stuffed Mushrooms

Serves 24	
Per serving:	
Calories:	30.98
Protein:	1.92 g
Carbohydrates:	2.63 g
Total fat:	1.65 g
Sat. fat:	0.68 g
Cholesterol:	2.69 mg
Sodium:	42.80 mg
Fiber:	0.49 g

24 large button mushrooms
Spectrum Naturals Extra Virgin
   Olive Spray Oil with Garlic
   Flavor
1 large sweet onion, chopped
1 large tomato, peeled, seeded,
   and chopped
1 green bell pepper, seeded and
   minced
2 teaspoons fresh lemon juice
1 tablespoon extra-virgin olive oil

⅛ teaspoon freshly ground black
   pepper
⅛ teaspoon mustard powder
1 teaspoon Italian Spice Blend
   (page 276)
¼ cup shredded provolone cheese
¼ cup shredded whole-milk
   mozzarella cheese
¼ cup grated Parmesan cheese
½ cup bread crumbs

1. Preheat oven to 400°.
2. Remove and chop the stems from the mushrooms; set aside. Lightly mist the tops and bottoms of the mushroom caps with the spray oil. Arrange in an oven-safe casserole dish or roasting pan, stem-side up.
3. Put the chopped mushroom stems, onion, tomato, green pepper, and lemon juice in a microwave-safe bowl. Cover and microwave on high for 3 to 5 minutes or until the onion is tender and transparent. Set aside to cool.
4. Stir the olive oil, pepper, mustard powder, Italian Blend, cheeses, and bread crumbs into the onion mixture. Evenly divide the mixture between the mushroom caps. Lightly mist the stuffed mushroom caps with the spray oil. Bake for 20 to 25 minutes or until the mushrooms are tender and the cheese is melted and bubbling.

Greek Yogurt Dip

1 cup nonfat plain yogurt
1 tablespoon fresh lemon juice
1 tablespoon granulated sugar
2 teaspoons Greek Spice Blend
   (page 277)

Add all the ingredients to a small bowl and mix well. Cover and refrigerate overnight to allow the flavors to intensify. Stir again before serving.

❁ Spice It Up

Using a mortar and pestle or spice grinder to process dried spices and herbs immediately before adding them to a recipe helps release their natural oils and flavors. An alternative to keep in mind is hand-cranked grinders—they aren't just for peppercorns anymore. Storing frequently used seasonings in a grinder provides a handy way to add ground herbs and spices to a recipe. For example, Oxo ceramic grinders are available individually or in sets filled with herbs like rosemary and spices like whole cloves.

Serves 16	
Per serving:	
Calories:	11.21
Protein:	0.82 g
Carbohydrates:	1.95 g
Total fat:	0.03 g
Sat. fat:	0.02 g
Cholesterol:	0.28 mg
Sodium:	10.94 mg
Fiber:	0.00 g

CHAPTER 2
Soups

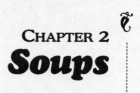

He-Man Serving-Size Gumbo

Serves 6	
Per serving:	
Calories:	458.17
Protein:	35.51 g
Carbohydrates:	61.00 g
Total fat:	7.58 g
Sat. fat:	1.47 g
Cholesterol:	130.88 mg
Sodium:	392.99 mg
Fiber:	6.30 g

1 tablespoon canola oil
1 large green bell pepper, chopped
1 cup finely chopped celery
1 large sweet onion, chopped
1 teaspoon freshly ground black pepper
2 teaspoons garlic powder
1 teaspoon Cajun Spice Blend (page 274)
1 tablespoon Old Bay Seasoning (page 274)
Optional: 1 tablespoon filé powder
5 cups water
¼ teaspoon Minor's Bacon Base
¼ teaspoon Minor's Ham Base
¾ teaspoon Minor's Low Sodium Beef Base
2 teaspoons Minor's Low Sodium Chicken Base
½ teaspoon Minor's Seafood Base
1 (14½-ounce) can Muir Glen Organic No Salt Added Diced Tomatoes
1 (10-ounce) package frozen sliced okra
¼ cup cornstarch
Optional: Mrs. Dash Extra Spicy Seasoning Blend or low-sodium hot sauce
¾ pound chicken breast, cooked and cut into pieces
¾ pound shrimp, peeled (or big shrimp, cut into pieces)
6 cups cooked brown rice

1. In a large, heavy nonstick skillet, heat the oil on medium-high. Add the green pepper and celery; sauté, stirring occasionally, for 3 minutes or until the celery begins to soften. Add the onion; sauté until the onion becomes transparent, about 5 minutes. Add the pepper, garlic powder, Cajun and Old Bay seasonings, and filé powder (if using it); stir.
2. Push the cooked vegetables to the side and add 1 cup of the water. Bring the water to a boil and add all the Minor's bases, whisking to dissolve.
3. Add 3½ cups of the remaining water, the tomatoes, and okra; bring to a boil. Stir the cornstarch into the remaining ½ cup of cold water; whisk the mixture into the gumbo along with the Mrs. Dash (if using).
4. Reduce heat and add the cooked chicken. Cover and simmer on low heat for 1 hour. Taste and adjust seasoning, if necessary. Add the shrimp and simmer until the shrimp turns pink. Serve over brown rice.

Oriental Tuna-Mushroom Soup

5 cups water
1 ounce dried whole shiitake
    mushrooms
½ teaspoon Bragg Liquid Aminos
1 teaspoon honey
2 cups fresh button mushrooms,
    sliced
2 teaspoons Minor's Low Sodium
    Chicken Base

4 teaspoons organic miso (yellow,
    shinshu miso)
2 slices peeled ginger
4 (¼") slices soft, silken tofu
1 (6-ounce) can Chicken of the Sea
    Very Low Sodium Tuna, drained
4 large green scallions, white and
    green part finely chopped

Serves 4	
Per serving:	
Calories:	145.51
Protein:	16.15 g
Carbohydrates:	14.51 g
Total fat:	3.70 g
Sat. fat:	0.60 g
Cholesterol:	16.23 mg
Sodium:	361.55 mg
Fiber:	2.72 g

1. In a saucepan or tea kettle, bring the water to a boil. Place the dried mushrooms in a bowl and pour enough boiling water over them to cover generously; set aside.

2. Add about ½ cup of the boiling water to a large, heavy nonstick skillet. Stir in the Bragg Liquid Aminos and honey. Add the sliced fresh mushrooms to the skillet, cover, and simmer on medium-low until tender, about 2 minutes. Remove from heat and set aside.

3. Use a slotted spoon to remove the reconstituted dried mushrooms from the water. Add the mushrooms to the skillet with the fresh mushrooms. Strain the liquid from the dried mushrooms to remove any sediment.

4. In another saucepan, whisk together the remaining water and the strained mushroom liquid with the chicken base, miso, and ginger. Bring to a simmer over medium heat for 5 minutes. Remove the ginger and keep the liquid hot.

5. To serve, place a slice of the tofu in each of 4 warmed soup bowls and top with the cooked mushrooms and tuna. Evenly ladle the chicken broth-miso soup on top and garnish with the chopped scallions.

Cream of Wild Mushroom Soup

Serves 4	
Per serving:	
Calories:	151.02
Protein:	7.18 g
Carbohydrates:	20.70 g
Total fat:	5.58 g
Sat. fat:	1.46 g
Cholesterol:	5.02 mg
Sodium:	245.12 mg
Fiber:	1.98 g

1 tablespoon olive oil
1 teaspoon unsalted butter
1 cup finely chopped shallots
2 cloves garlic, minced
2 cups thinly sliced button mushrooms
2 cups thinly sliced mixed fresh
  wild mushrooms
2 tablespoons unbleached all-purpose flour

5 cups water
3 teaspoons Minor's Low Sodium
  Chicken Base
½ cup instant nonfat dry milk
Optional: Freshly ground nutmeg
Optional: Freshly ground black
  pepper
¼ cup chopped fresh parsley

1. In a large, heavy nonstick skillet, heat the oil and melt the butter over medium-high heat. Add the shallots and garlic; cook, stirring, for 1 minute. Add the mushrooms; sauté until the mushrooms become soft and most of the mushroom liquid is evaporated, about 8 minutes.
2. Sprinkle flour over the mushroom mixture and stir well to make a roux, cooking for about 2 minutes.
3. Gradually whisk in the water. Raise the temperature and bring to a boil. Whisk in the chicken base until dissolved.
4. Reduce heat and simmer for about 20 minutes, stirring frequently.
5. Whisk in the nonfat dry milk until dissolved.
6. Ladle into soup bowls and garnish with freshly ground nutmeg, pepper, and chopped parsley.

Caribbean-Seasoned Puréed Vegetable Soup

1 tablespoon canola or grapeseed oil

1 large sweet onion, diced

2 cloves garlic, minced

1 large stalk celery, diced

½ teaspoon dried ginger

¼ teaspoon ground mustard

⅛ teaspoon allspice

½ teaspoon hot paprika

¼ teaspoon dried thyme

⅛ teaspoon fennel seed, crushed

⅛ teaspoon dried ground cloves

¼ teaspoon cayenne

¼ teaspoon freshly ground black pepper

4 carrots, peeled and diced

3 large potatoes, peeled and diced

1 medium-sized sweet potato, peeled and diced

2 leeks, white part only, washed well and diced

2 teaspoons Minor's Low Sodium Chicken Base

4 cups water

½ cup smooth no-salt-added peanut butter

½ cup tahini

Optional: Minced fresh parsley, for garnish

Optional: Dried red pepper flakes, for garnish

Optional: Chopped scallions, for garnish

Serves 6	
Per serving:	
Calories:	462.25
Protein:	13.42 g
Carbohydrates:	55.53 g
Total fat:	23.56 g
Sat. fat:	3.94 g
Cholesterol:	0.40 mg
Sodium:	125.87 mg
Fiber:	8.19 g

1. In a large saucepan, heat the oil and sauté the onions, garlic, and celery, stirring until the onions are transparent.
2. Add the spices and sauté for 1 minute.
3. Add the carrots, potatoes, leeks, base, and water. Bring the soup to a boil; reduce the heat, cover, and simmer until the vegetables are tender, about 25 minutes.
4. Use a hand blender to stir in the peanut butter and tahini and to purée the vegetables. (Alternatively, transfer the soup to a blender or food processor to purée it.) Garnish with the optional ingredients, if desired, and serve.

Pumpkin and Ginger Soup

Serves 4	
Per serving:	
Calories:	82.73
Protein:	1.60 g
Carbohydrates:	12.24 g
Total fat:	3.74 g
Sat. fat:	0.32 g
Cholesterol:	0.00 mg
Sodium:	46.15 mg
Fiber:	2.50 g

1 tablespoon canola or grapeseed oil
1 medium-sized sweet onion, sliced
1 large stalk celery, sliced
2 bay leaves
¼ teaspoon dried thyme
¼ teaspoon dried oregano
4 carrots, sliced
2 cups pumpkin, cut into 1" cubes

3 tablespoons minced fresh ginger
4 cups water
Optional: ½ teaspoon cinnamon
Optional: Pinch each of ground cloves, allspice, and mace
Optional: Freshly ground black pepper, to taste

1. In a large saucepan, heat the oil and sauté the onions and celery, stirring until the onions are transparent.
2. Add the bay leaves, thyme, oregano, carrots, pumpkin, ginger, and water; bring to a boil. Reduce heat, cover, and simmer until the vegetables are tender, about 25 minutes.
3. Remove and discard the bay leaves. Use a hand blender to purée the soup. (Alternatively, transfer the soup to a blender or food processor to purée it.) Serve warm, sprinkled with cinnamon, optional spices, and freshly ground black pepper, if desired.

❄ Flavor Enhancing 101

A tablespoon of dry white wine or vermouth per serving is an excellent, low-sodium way to punch up the flavor of soup. Just be sure to add it to the soup during the cooking process to allow enough time for the alcohol to evaporate.

Quick Lean Beef Stew

1 teaspoon olive oil

1 medium-sized sweet or white onion, diced

1 large stalk celery, chopped

1 (8-ounce) boneless sirloin steak, thinly sliced against the grain

2 cloves garlic, minced

¼ teaspoon freshly ground black pepper

⅛ teaspoon dried orange or lemon peel granules, crushed

Pinch ground cloves

4 medium-sized potatoes, peeled and diced

1 (14.5-ounce) can Muir Glen Organic No Salt Added Diced Tomatoes

3 cups water

1½ teaspoons Minor's Low Sodium Beef Base

1 (10-ounce) bag Cascadian Farm Gardener's Blend frozen vegetables

Optional: 1 tablespoon Maple Leaf Potato Granules (or other non-seasoned, no-fat-added instant mashed potato flakes or potato flour)

Serves 4	
Per serving:	
Calories:	345.37
Protein:	20.95 g
Carbohydrates:	50.92 g
Total fat:	6.67 g
Sat. fat:	2.31 g
Cholesterol:	44.73 mg
Sodium:	191.92 mg
Fiber:	6.96 g

1. In a large, deep nonstick sauté pan, heat the olive oil over medium-high heat and add the onion and celery; sauté until the onion is almost transparent.
2. Add the thinly sliced beef, minced garlic, pepper, citrus peel, and ground cloves; stir-fry until the beef is lightly browned.
3. Add the potatoes, tomatoes, and water; bring to a boil. Add the beef base and stir to dissolve. Lower the heat, cover, and simmer until the potatoes are tender, about 15 minutes.
4. Add the frozen vegetable blend. Bring back to simmer and cook until the vegetables are heated through, about 5 minutes.
5. For a thicker stew, mix potato granules with 2 to 4 tablespoons of water or broth from the stew, stirring well to stir out any lumps. Add to the stew. Mix well, stirring until the stew thickens. Serve immediately.

Pepper Pot Soup

Serves 4	
Per serving:	
Calories:	285.41
Protein:	12.89 g
Carbohydrates:	47.84 g
Total fat:	5.35 g
Sat. fat:	1.49 g
Cholesterol:	22.64 mg
Sodium:	216.58 mg
Fiber:	6.34 g

2 teaspoons olive oil
1 medium-sized sweet onion, chopped
Optional: 1 leek, cleaned and chopped
Optional: 1 green onion, cleaned and chopped
Optional: 1 shallot, cleaned and chopped
1 large green bell pepper, cleaned, seeded, and chopped
¼ teaspoon dried thyme
¼ teaspoon dried marjoram
¼ teaspoon ground cloves

Pinch dried red pepper flakes
½ teaspoon freshly ground black pepper
4-ounce boneless sirloin steak, thinly sliced against the grain, then cut into small pieces
¼ teaspoon Minor's Ham Base
¼ teaspoon Minor's Bacon Base
1 teaspoon Minor's Low Sodium Beef Base
4 medium-sized potatoes, peeled and diced
1 bay leaf
4 cups water

1. In a large, deep nonstick sauté pan, heat the oil over medium heat. Add the chopped onion, green pepper, and the leek, green onion, and shallot (if using); sauté until the onion is transparent.
2. Add the thyme, marjoram, cloves, red pepper flakes, and black pepper. Stir to mix with the green peppers and onions. Push the vegetables to the side of the pan and add the beef; stir-fry for 2 minutes.
3. Add the Minor's bases and stir to dissolve. Add the potatoes; stir and lightly sauté in the onion-beef mixture for about 1 minute.
4. Add the bay leaf and water; bring to a boil. Reduce heat, cover, and simmer for 20 minutes or until the potatoes are tender. Remove and discard the bay leaf before serving. Optional step: For a thicker soup, use a hand blender to cream the soup. The starch from the potatoes acts as a natural roux (without adding the fat and calories of a roux made with butter and flour). Serve warm garnished with an additional grind of freshly ground black pepper on top.

Baked Potato Soup

1 (16-ounce) bag frozen Cascadian
Farm Country Style Potatoes
½ cup shredded sharp Cheddar
cheese
¼ teaspoon Minor's Bacon Base
¼ teaspoon Minor's Ham Base
½ teaspoon Minor's Low Sodium
Chicken Base

¼ cup nonfat yogurt
¼ cup instant nonfat dry milk
1 cup Garlic Broth (page 33)
¼ cup Herb Broth (page 32)
2½ cups water
Freshly ground pepper, to taste
Optional: Fresh chives, snipped

Serves 4	
Per serving:	
Calories:	177.92
Protein:	9.20 g
Carbohydrates:	26.31 g
Total fat:	5.03 g
Sat. fat:	3.13 g
Cholesterol:	16.26 mg
Sodium:	289.50 mg
Fiber:	5.37 g

1. Preheat oven to 350°.
2. Treat a deep (3-quart or larger) Pyrex casserole dish with nonstick
   spray. Spread the frozen potatoes over the bottom of the pan. Cover
   with microwave-safe plastic wrap and microwave for 3 minutes at 50
   percent power to defrost the potato mixture. Remove and discard the
   plastic wrap. Top with the cheese.
3. In a blender or food processor, combine the bases, yogurt, dry milk,
   broths, and water; pulse until well-mixed. Pour the mixture over the
   cheese and potatoes. Bake for 45 minutes or until the cheese is
   melted and bubbly. Sprinkle with the freshly ground pepper and
   snipped chives, if desired, and serve.

❀ Substitution Simplicity

*Omitting the salt called for in recipes is the best way to reduce the
sodium in your diet. If you're afraid to go "cold turkey," try substituting mustard powder for the salt. The rule of thumb is to use
¼ teaspoon mustard powder for every 4 servings. Later, if you
insist, season the food with a little sea salt at the table. Once you
get in that habit, you'll find that it takes far less salt than you
thought to enhance the flavors of food!*

Quick Hearty Vegetable Soup

Serves 4	
Per serving:	
Calories:	229.52
Protein:	13.15 g
Carbohydrates:	33.12 g
Total fat:	5.69 g
Sat. fat:	2.96 g
Cholesterol:	13.91 mg
Sodium:	215.64 mg
Fiber:	12.02 g

1 teaspoon corn or canola oil
1 large sweet onion, chopped
1 clove garlic, finely chopped
½ teaspoon (or more, to taste) salt-free red chili powder
1 teaspoon ancho chili powder
¼ teaspoon ground cumin
¼ teaspoon ground coriander
1 tablespoon unsweetened, no-salt-added applesauce
1 teaspoon Minor's Low Sodium Chicken Base
1 (15-ounce) can Eden Organic No Salt Added Kidney Beans
1 bay leaf
⅛ teaspoon dried oregano
¼ teaspoon dried basil
1 (14.5-ounce) can Muir Glen Organic No Salt Added Diced Tomatoes
2 cups water
1 (10-ounce) bag Cascadian Farm Gardener's Blend frozen vegetables
½ cup grated Monterey jack or Muenster cheese
½ bunch cilantro leaves, roughly chopped
Optional: Whole cilantro leaves, for garnish

1. Heat the oil in a large, deep nonstick sauté pan treated with nonstick spray; sauté the onions over high heat for 1 to 2 minutes. Lower the heat and stir in the garlic, chili powders, cumin, and coriander; sauté until the garlic is tender. Add the applesauce and chicken base; mix well to dissolve the chicken base.
2. Add the beans, bay leaf, oregano, basil, tomatoes, water, and frozen vegetables. Simmer until the vegetables are cooked, about 15 to 20 minutes.
3. Stir in the cheese and chopped cilantro. Garnish with whole leaves of cilantro, if desired. Serve with cornbread or tortillas.

Quick Thick Peanut Soup

½ cup creamy no-salt-added
   peanut butter
1 teaspoon onion powder
1 teaspoon dried celery flakes
Pinch dried red pepper flakes
1 teaspoon Minor's Low Sodium
   Chicken Base
¼ teaspoon Minor's Ham Base

3 cups water
¼ cup instant nonfat dry milk
½ cup Maple Leaf Potato Granules
   (or other unseasoned, no-salt-
   added instant potato flakes or
   potato flour)

Serves 4	
Per serving:	
Calories:	282.15
Protein:	11.95 g
Carbohydrates:	25.19 g
Total fat:	16.73 g
Sat. fat:	3.46 g
Cholesterol:	1.13 mg
Sodium:	155.04 mg
Fiber:	2.90 g

1. Heat the peanut butter in a nonstick saucepan over medium heat.
   Add the onion powder, celery flakes, dried peppers, and bases,
   stirring constantly until the bases are dissolved and well mixed.
2. In a blender or food processor, combine the water, dry milk, and
   potato granules; process until blended.
3. Slowly pour the water mixture into the peanut butter, whisking to
   combine. Lower the heat and simmer until the mixture is heated
   through and thickened, stirring gently. Serve immediately.

❀ Compost Broth

*This isn't as yucky as it sounds. Rather, it's a frugal way to use
the peelings from vegetables that you'd probably otherwise just
throw away. Instead, wash vegetables before you peel them and
place the peelings in a 1-gallon sealable plastic bag. Store the bag
in the refrigerator for a few days until you've got enough peelings
and you're ready to make the broth. Include stuff you'd usually
never dream of using, like onion and garlic peel! Simmer the peelings in at least 1 gallon of water for 1 hour. Strain the broth, and
voilà! You have veggie broth.*

Chilled Cucumber Soup

Serves 4	
Per serving:	
Calories:	62.55
Protein:	3.84 g
Carbohydrates:	9.94 g
Total fat:	1.03 g
Sat. fat:	0.56 g
Cholesterol:	3.68 mg
Sodium:	100.24 mg
Fiber:	0.98 g

2 large cucumbers, peeled, seeded, and chopped
1 tablespoon Cascadian Farm frozen Organic Apple Juice Concentrate
1 tablespoon Spectrum Naturals Red Wine Vinegar
1½ cups cold, cultured low-fat buttermilk
Optional: Dried dill weed
Optional: Lemon zest

1. Place the cucumbers, apple juice concentrate, and vinegar in a food processor. Process briefly, then add the buttermilk and process again until smooth.
2. Cover and refrigerate until ready to serve. Serve chilled with a pinch of dried dill weed and some lemon zest floating on top of each serving, if desired.

Butternut Squash Soup

Serves 4	
Per serving:	
Calories:	120.00
Protein:	3.00 g
Carbohydrates:	30.00 g
Total fat:	1.00 g
Sat. fat:	0.00 g
Cholesterol:	0.00 mg
Sodium:	290.00 mg
Fiber:	8.00 g

¼ teaspoon extra-virgin olive oil
4 cups diced, peeled butternut squash
1 large yellow onion, chopped
4 stalks celery, chopped
1 bay leaf
2 teaspoons dried oregano
¼ teaspoon ground nutmeg
⅓ teaspoon salt
¼ teaspoon freshly ground black pepper
4 cups vegetable stock

1. Heat the olive oil in a stockpot over medium heat. Add the squash, onion, and celery; sauté until the onion has softened, about 2 minutes. Add the bay leaf, oregano, nutmeg, salt, and pepper; sauté for an additional 2 minutes.
2. Add the stock and bring to a boil. Reduce heat and simmer until the squash is soft, about 20 to 25 minutes.
3. If desired, use a hand blender to cream the soup. Serve warm.

Cocoa in Black Bean Soup

1 teaspoon peanut or canola oil
1 small sweet onion, minced
1 large green bell pepper, cored and diced
2 cloves garlic, minced
¼ teaspoon freshly ground black pepper
¼ teaspoon dried ground ancho pepper (or salt-free chili powder)
⅛ teaspoon ground cumin
⅛ teaspoon cinnamon
2 teaspoons unsweetened cocoa powder
1 tablespoon American Spoon Foods jalapeño jelly
1 cup water
1 (15-ounce) can Eden Organic No Salt Added Black Beans
4 teaspoons Spectrum Naturals Red Wine Vinegar
4 teaspoons extra-virgin olive oil
Optional: No-salt-added peanut or almond butter

Serves 4	
Per serving:	
Calories:	154.28
Protein:	6.28 g
Carbohydrates:	20.09 g
Total fat:	5.80 g
Sat. fat:	0.88 g
Cholesterol:	0.00 mg
Sodium:	15.88 mg
Fiber:	5.55 g

1. In a large, deep nonstick sauté pan, heat the oil on medium. Add the onion and green pepper; sauté until tender.
2. Add the garlic, black pepper, ancho pepper or chili powder, cumin, cinnamon, and cocoa; stir well, slightly sautéing the spices. Stir in the jalapeño jelly until dissolved.
3. Add the water and black beans. Bring to serving temperature over medium-low heat. Just prior to serving, add the red wine vinegar and olive oil, and stir well.
4. Divide into serving bowls and serve warm. If desired, serve peanut or almond butter at the table for those who want to add it to their soup.

Peanut Butter Power

Many health food stores carry fresh-ground peanut butter. Once you taste peanut butter made fresh from dry-roasted nuts, you won't miss the salt, sugar, and other extra stuff that is added to commercial brands.

Herb Broth

Serves 32	
Per serving:	
Calories:	1.53
Protein:	0.04 g
Carbohydrates:	0.36 g
Total fat:	0.00 g
Sat. fat:	0.00 g
Cholesterol:	0.00 mg
Sodium:	0.09 mg
Fiber:	0.04 g

¼ cup dried thyme
¼ cup dried parsley
¼ cup dried minced onion
2 tablespoons dried oregano
20 black peppercorns
8 bay leaves

1 teaspoon dried lavender
Optional: 1 teaspoon dried lemon
thyme or dried lemon peel
granules
9 cups boiling water

1. Place all the ingredients *except* the water in a stockpot. Bring the water to a boil in a separate pot.
2. Pour at least 2 cups of boiling water over the dried ingredients in the stockpot. (Pouring boiling water over the dried herbs more effectively releases the flavors than does bringing them to a boil in cold water.) Let sit for a few minutes. Add the remaining water to the stockpot and bring to a boil; reduce heat and simmer, uncovered, for 1 hour.
3. Pour the broth through a fine-mesh strainer. Add additional water, if necessary, to yield a total of 8 cups of broth. Refrigerate until needed, up to 3 days. You can also freeze the broth in 1-cup portions so it's easily available to add to recipes. (Another alternative is to make broth cubes. Most ice cube sections hold 2 tablespoons of liquid per cube, so 8 broth cubes will equal 1 cup of broth.)

❈ Pork Broth

Pork broth is seldom called for in recipes, but it can add a wonderful additional layer of flavor when mixed with chicken broth in bean or vegetable soups. Once the meat has been removed from the resulting broth in the Easy Slow-Cooked Pork recipe (page 152), strain the broth; once cooled, cover and refrigerate the broth overnight. Remove and discard the hardened fat. The broth can be kept for 1 or 2 days in the refrigerator, or frozen up to 3 months. On average, the nutritional analysis for each ½-cup serving of the resulting pork broth will be: Calories: 33.48; Protein: 2.31 g; Carbohydrates: 0.32 g; Total Fat: 2.50 g; Sat. Fat: 0.89 g; Cholesterol: 8.98 mg; Sodium: 148.95 mg; Fiber: 0.00 g.

Garlic Broth

9 cups water
4 cloves garlic, crushed
2 carrots, peeled and chopped
2 stalks celery, chopped

1 small sweet onion, quartered
5 black peppercorns
1 bay leaf

Serves 8	
Per serving:	
Calories:	9.19
Protein:	0.31 g
Carbohydrates:	2.10 g
Total fat:	0.04 g
Sat. fat:	0.01 g
Cholesterol:	0.00 mg
Sodium:	8.56 mg
Fiber:	0.08 g

1. In a stockpot, bring the water to a boil. Add the remaining ingredients. Reduce the heat, cover, and simmer for 1 hour.
2. Pour the resulting stock through a strainer, pressing as much liquid as possible from the cooked vegetables.
3. Cool the stock and refrigerate until needed, up to 3 days. Alternatively, freeze the broth in 1-cup portions so it's easily available to add to recipes. (Another alternative is to make broth cubes. Most ice cube sections hold 2 tablespoons of liquid per cube, so 8 broth cubes will equal 1 cup of broth.)

❀ Cholesterol Facts

A study published in the New England Journal of Medicine in 1990 said studies revealed conclusive evidence that transfatty acids increase cholesterol—the low-density lipoprotein (LDL) that contributes to cardiovascular disease. Watch out for margarine that contains transfatty acids; while it may be labeled as cholesterol-free, it actually encourages the production of bad cholesterol in the body. (Most commercially prepared white bread is high in transfatty acids, too.)

Za'atar Meatball Stew

Serves 8	
Per serving:	
Calories:	260.32
Protein:	21.39 g
Carbohydrates:	35.52 g
Total fat:	4.50 g
Sat. fat:	1.32 g
Cholesterol:	33.30 mg
Sodium:	184.29 mg
Fiber:	8.80 g

½ pound lean ground chicken or turkey
½ pound lean ground sirloin or round
1 large sweet onion, diced
1 large red bell pepper, seeded and diced
1 large green bell pepper, seeded and diced
½ teaspoon freshly ground black pepper
1 tablespoon (or more, to taste) za'atar
1 teaspoon ground cumin

¼ teaspoon brown sugar
1 (28-ounce) can Muir Glen Organic Tomato Purée
1 (14.5-ounce) can Muir Glen Organic Stewed Tomatoes
1 (15-ounce) can Eden Organic No Salt Added Black Beans
1 (15-ounce) can Eden Organic Chickpeas
Optional: Cooked brown rice or whole-grain noodles
Optional: Plain nonfat yogurt
Optional: Fresh mint or parsley

1. Preheat oven to 300°.
2. Mix together the ground chicken (or turkey) and beef. Form into 16 small (tablespoon-size) meatballs.
3. In a deep, nonstick, oven-safe Dutch oven treated with nonstick spray, sauté the meatballs until browned. Remove the meatballs with a slotted spoon. Sauté the onion and bell peppers in the fat from the meat for about 3 minutes, until tender.
4. Add the pepper, za'atar, cumin, and brown sugar; sauté for 1 minute, stirring to mix with the onion and peppers. Add the tomato purée, stewed tomatoes, beans, and chickpeas; stir well and bring the mixture to temperature. (Taste the tomato mixture and add more za'atar and black pepper, if desired.) Add the meatballs to the tomato mixture. Transfer the Dutch oven to the preheated oven and bake for 1½ hours.
5. Serve over cooked brown rice or whole-grain noodles and garnish with a dollop of plain nonfat yogurt and a sprig of mint or parsley, if desired.

Borscht

1 tablespoon olive oil
1 teaspoon unsalted butter
1 large sweet onion, chopped
2 teaspoons Minor's Low Sodium
   Beef Base
6 cups water
1 (28-ounce) can Muir Glen
   Organic Whole Peeled Tomatoes
   with juice, coarsely chopped
1 pound beets, peeled and cut in
   ¼" slices

1 small head cabbage, cored and
   shredded
3 carrots, peeled and sliced
3 parsnips, peeled and chopped
3 bay leaves
1 tablespoon caraway seeds
½ teaspoon ground allspice
2 tablespoons red wine vinegar
Optional: Plain nonfat yogurt

Serves 8	
Per serving:	
Calories:	144.21
Protein:	3.39 g
Carbohydrates:	28.93 g
Total fat:	2.82 g
Sat. fat:	0.69 g
Cholesterol:	1.70 mg
Sodium:	305.80 mg
Fiber:	5.96 g

1. In a pressure cooker, heat the olive oil and butter on medium. Add the onions and sauté until soft, stirring frequently for about 3 minutes. Add all the remaining ingredients *except* the vinegar and yogurt.
2. Lock the lid of the pressure cooker in place. Bring to high pressure over high heat. Adjust the heat to maintain high pressure, and cook for 10 minutes. Remove from heat and let the pressure drop naturally or, to quick-release the pressure, place the pot under cold, running water. (Other quick-release methods are likely to cause sputtering.)
3. Remove the lid, tilting it away from you to allow any excess steam to escape. Remove and discard the bay leaves. Stir in the vinegar. Serve warm, garnishing each portion with a dollop of plain nonfat yogurt, if desired.

❀ Borscht Basics
Although borscht is traditionally made with beef stock, it's easy to make a vegetarian version by substituting a full-flavored vegetable stock.

Pork and Sauerkraut Soup

Serves 8	
Per serving:	
Calories:	411.38
Protein:	28.28 g
Carbohydrates:	35.63 g
Total fat:	16.79 g
Sat. fat:	5.41 g
Cholesterol:	72.67 mg
Sodium:	465.92 mg
Fiber:	8.05 g

2 pounds lean, boneless pork roast, cut in 1" cubes
1 teaspoon granulated sugar
2 teaspoons Hungarian paprika
1 teaspoon freshly ground black pepper
1 tablespoon olive oil
1 stalk celery, sliced
1 large sweet onion, diced
3 cloves garlic, minced
1 tablespoon fresh lemon juice
¼ teaspoon Minor's Ham Base

¼ teaspoon Minor's Bacon Base
1 bay leaf
2 cups water
2 carrots, peeled and sliced
2 large potatoes, peeled and diced
1 (15-ounce) can no-salt-added pinto beans
1 (24-ounce) jar Muir Glen Organic Reduced-Sodium Sauerkraut, drained
Optional: Plain nonfat yogurt

1. Season the pork with the sugar, paprika, and pepper. Heat the oil in a pressure cooker on medium-high. Add the pork and brown it, searing the meat on all sides. Remove the meat with a slotted spoon and set aside.

2. Add the celery to the pressure cooker and sauté for 1 minute. Add the onion and sauté until the onion is transparent, about 5 more minutes. Add the garlic and sauté for 1 more minute. Add the lemon juice and Minor's bases, stirring to dissolve the bases.

3. Add the pork back to the pressure cooker. Add the bay leaf, water, carrots, and potatoes. Place the lid on the pressure cooker and bring it up to 15 pounds of pressure. Maintain pressure and cook for 15 minutes.

4. Quick-cool the cooker by running cool tap water over the lid. Remove the lid and test the carrots and potatoes; they should be fork tender. Add the beans and sauerkraut. Stir to mix and bring to temperature over medium heat. (If additional cooking time is needed for the carrots and potatoes, cover and simmer the soup for 5 to 10 minutes.)

5. Serve warm. Garnish each serving with a dollop of plain nonfat yogurt topped with additional freshly ground black pepper and Hungarian paprika, if desired.

Oven Beef Stew

1 tablespoon olive oil
2 pounds lean, boneless sirloin
   roast, cut into 1" cubes
½ pound lean ground pork
¼ teaspoon Minor's Bacon or
   Ham Base
1 teaspoon high-bulk-index granulated garlic powder
1 teaspoon paprika
½ teaspoon freshly ground pepper
¼ teaspoon thyme
⅛ teaspoon ground ginger
⅛ teaspoon ground cinnamon
⅛ teaspoon ground cloves
⅛ teaspoon dried oregano
⅛ teaspoon mustard powder
2 medium-sized sweet onions, chopped
1 stalk celery, sliced
Optional: 1 cup sliced mushrooms

1 cup hearty red wine
Pinch dried red pepper flakes or
   a dash of hot sauce
1 (14.5-ounce) can Muir Glen
   Organic No Salt Added
   Chopped Tomatoes
5 medium-sized Yukon gold potatoes, peeled and cubed
5 carrots, peeled and sliced
2 cups water
½ cup low-salt ketchup
1 (10-ounce) package frozen
   Cascadian Farm Petite Sweet Peas
1 (10-ounce) package frozen
   Cascadian Farm Super Sweet Corn
1 (10-ounce) package frozen
   Cascadian Farm Whole Green
   Beans

Serves 10	
Per serving:	
Calories:	461.40
Protein:	36.56 g
Carbohydrates:	40.21 g
Total fat:	15.64 g
Sat. fat:	5.62 g
Cholesterol:	97.13 mg
Sodium:	180.45 mg
Fiber:	6.04 g

1. Preheat oven to 300°.
2. In a large ovenproof Dutch oven, heat the oil on medium-high. Brown the sirloin pieces in the pan in 3 separate batches (do not crowd the pan), stirring often and removing each batch before adding more.
3. Add the ground pork to the pan. Add the Minor's base, garlic powder, paprika, pepper, thyme, ginger, cinnamon, cloves, oregano, and mustard powder; mix well to combine with the meat. Sauté the pork for 2 minutes, then add the onion and celery. Continue to sauté until the onion is transparent. Push to the side of the pan and add the mushrooms, sautéing until tender and the moisture releases from the mushrooms.

(continues on page 38)

Oven Beef Stew
(continued)

4. Add the red wine and cook over medium-high heat for 2 minutes to evaporate the alcohol, stirring well and scraping the bottom of the Dutch oven to loosen browned meat bits. Add the red pepper flakes (or hot sauce), tomatoes, potatoes, sliced carrots, water, and ketchup; stir well.

5. Cover the pan with foil or an ovenproof lid. Bake for 3 hours. (No additional stirring is necessary during that time.)

6. Remove from the oven and place the pan over low heat. Carefully remove the lid. Add the frozen vegetables. Stir to combine and simmer for 20 to 30 minutes to heat the vegetables and concentrate the sauce.

❁ Seasoning Swaps

High-bulk-index granulated garlic is available from the Spice House (see Appendix B) and other specialty spice outlets. You can substitute 2 to 3 teaspoons dried minced garlic or regular garlic powder instead. Another delicious change of pace is to add 1 or 2 teaspoons of additional seasoning, such as the Spice House's Salt-Free Bavarian Style Seasoning or the Spice Hunter's Salt-Free Natural Hickory Barbecue Blend.

Speedy Jambalaya

1 tablespoon olive oil

¼ teaspoon Minor's Ham Base

½ pound lean pork roast, cut into 1" cubes

½ pound boneless chicken breast, cut into 1" cubes

4 stalks celery, sliced

1 large green bell pepper, seeded and chopped

2 cups coarsely chopped white onion

4 cloves garlic, minced

¼ teaspoon dried thyme

½ teaspoon dried basil

1 teaspoon dried parsley

1¼ cups uncooked long-grain brown rice

2 cups water

1 bay leaf

2 tablespoons Muir Glen Organic No Salt Added Tomato Paste

Pinch dried red pepper

1 tablespoon fresh lemon juice

Serves 4	
Per serving:	
Calories:	436.01
Protein:	33.23 g
Carbohydrates:	49.67 g
Total fat:	10.93 g
Sat. fat:	2.70 g
Cholesterol:	81.71 mg
Sodium:	167.27 mg
Fiber:	3.05 g

1. Heat the oil in a pressure cooker on medium. Add the Minor's Ham Base and stir to combine with the oil. Brown the pork and chicken in 2 or 3 batches (do not crowd the pan), removing each batch with a slotted spoon before adding more. Set aside the browned meat.

2. Add the celery, green peppers, and onions; sauté for 3 minutes or until the onions are transparent. Add the garlic and sauté for 1 minute more.

3. Add the thyme, basil, parsley, and rice; sauté for about 1 minute, stirring well to coat the rice in the pan juices.

4. Add the water, bay leaf, tomato paste, and red pepper. Add the browned meat back to the pan and stir to combine.

5. Lock the lid in place and bring to high pressure over high heat. Maintain high pressure and cook for 15 minutes. Reduce the heat to low and let the pressure drop naturally for 10 minutes. Quick-release any remaining pressure by running cool tap water over the lid. Remove the lid. (If the rice is slightly undercooked, cover and simmer over low heat for another 2 or 3 minutes. Stir in a couple of tablespoons of water, if necessary.) Remove and discard the bay leaf and stir in the lemon juice before serving.

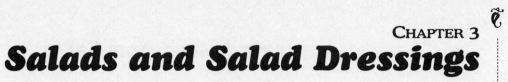

CHAPTER 3

Salads and Salad Dressings

Marinated Mushroom Salad

Serves 8	
Per serving:	
Calories:	88.10
Protein:	1.73 g
Carbohydrates:	5.24 g
Total fat:	7.40 g
Sat. fat:	0.97 g
Cholesterol:	0.00 mg
Sodium:	176.76 mg
Fiber:	1.67 g

2 cups small button mushroom caps
1 medium-sized zucchini, washed and cubed (peeling optional)
1 medium-sized yellow squash, washed and cubed (peeling optional)
¼ cup fresh lemon juice
¼ cup extra-virgin olive, grapeseed, avocado, walnut, or almond oil

½ teaspoon Dijon mustard
½ teaspoon mustard powder
1 teaspoon granulated sugar
½ teaspoon dried basil, crushed
¼ teaspoon freshly ground black pepper

1. Prepare the mushrooms, zucchini, and yellow squash. Put in a bowl large enough to allow the vegetables to be tossed with the vinaigrette marinade.
2. To prepare the marinade, combine the lemon juice, oil, mustard, sugar, basil, and pepper in a screw-top jar, cover, and shake well. Pour over the mushroom mixture.
3. Marinate, covered, in the refrigerator for 4 hours or overnight, tossing or stirring the mixture occasionally.

❀ Grapeseed Oil
Grapeseed oil has the highest smoke point of all oils. You can use it to replace peanut oil in stir-fry recipes. To treat baking sheets to be used at higher oven temperatures, Spectrum Naturals Grapeseed Spray Oil can be used instead of Spectrum Naturals Super Canola Spray Oil, if you prefer.

Tofu, Oil, and Vinegar Salad Dressing

1 tablespoon extra-virgin olive oil
2 tablespoons silken tofu
1 tablespoon vinegar

1 teaspoon ground mustard
Optional: Choice of herbs, spices,
 and freshly ground black pepper

Put all the ingredients in a small bowl and whisk to combine. Pour over your choice of prepared salad greens and vegetables.

Serves 4	
Per serving:	
Calories:	35.82
Protein:	0.57 g
Carbohydrates:	0.43 g
Total fat:	3.69 g
Sat. fat:	0.50 g
Cholesterol:	0.00 mg
Sodium:	0.61 mg
Fiber:	0.03 g

Zesty Corn Relish

4 banana or jalapeño peppers,
 stemmed, seeded, and chopped
⅓ cup frozen corn, thawed
⅓ cup chopped red onion
⅛ teaspoon Texas Seasoning
 (page 275)

2 teaspoons lime juice
Freshly ground black pepper

Combine all the ingredients in a bowl and toss to mix. This can be served immediately, or it can be chilled and served the next day.

Serves 4	
Per serving:	
Calories:	39.33
Protein:	1.64 g
Carbohydrates:	9.00 g
Total fat:	0.40 g
Sat. fat:	0.06 g
Cholesterol:	0.00 mg
Sodium:	6.57 mg
Fiber:	2.09 g

Roasted Shallot Vinaigrette

Serves 20	
Per serving:	
Calories:	109.26
Protein:	0.55 g
Carbohydrates:	1.58 g
Total fat:	11.57 g
Sat. fat:	1.72 g
Cholesterol:	1.04 mg
Sodium:	140.33 mg
Fiber:	0.40 g

2 teaspoons unsalted butter, melted
¼ cup chopped shallots
¼ cup cider vinegar
1½ tablespoons lemon juice
1 teaspoon Dijon mustard
1 cup extra-virgin olive oil

½ teaspoon fennel seeds, crushed
Freshly ground black pepper, to taste
Optional: 1 teaspoon Cascadian
   Farm frozen Organic Apple
   Juice Concentrate

1. Melt the butter in a sauté pan on medium heat. Add the shallots and sauté them, stirring or tossing them constantly to prevent them from burning. Sauté the shallots until they are caramelized (until they turn golden brown). Cool the shallots in the refrigerator.
2. Add the vinegar, lemon juice, mustard, olive oil, fennel seeds, and pepper to a covered jar. Shake well until the mixture is emulsified. (Alternatively, add the ingredients to a blender or a food processor and process until mixed.) Add the shallots and shake again.

❋ Pucker Up

Fruit and herb vinegars are usually flavored cider or wine vinegars. Experiment with using different varieties in your recipes. Sherry vinegar and champagne vinegar are two other choices; some people find that it takes less oil to offset their milder flavors. When a vinaigrette is too tart because of a strong vinegar, instead of adding more oil, try mixing in some frozen fruit juice concentrate, 1 teaspoon at a time.

Veggie-Fruit Salad

1 ripe avocado, peeled and pit removed

½ cup plain nonfat yogurt

1 tablespoon Hellmann's or Best Foods Real Mayonnaise

2 teaspoons lemon juice, divided

¼ teaspoon finely grated lime or lemon zest

1 tablespoon finely chopped fresh cilantro

1 tablespoon finely chopped fresh parsley

¼ teaspoon ground mustard

1 clove garlic, minced

4 scallions, white and green parts finely chopped

1 cup chopped poached chicken breast, unsalted

⅛ teaspoon freshly ground pepper

2 cups salad greens, torn into bite-size pieces

2 cups cubed cantaloupe

2 cups seedless green grapes

2 cups cherry tomatoes

1 cup diced celery

Serves 4	
Per serving:	
Calories:	286.29
Protein:	16.50 g
Carbohydrates:	34.74 g
Total fat:	11.29 g
Sat. fat:	2.06 g
Cholesterol:	31.32 mg
Sodium:	128.80 mg
Fiber:	6.31 g

1. In a small bowl, mash the avocado with a fork. Add the yogurt, mayonnaise, 1 teaspoon of the lemon juice, the zest, cilantro, parsley, ground mustard, garlic, and scallions; mix well.
2. In a large bowl, toss the chicken breast with the remaining teaspoon of lemon juice and the freshly ground black pepper. Add the salad greens, cantaloupe, grapes, cherry tomatoes, and celery; toss well. Divide the salad between 4 plates.
3. Divide the dressing between the 4 salads. Garnish with additional finely chopped cilantro or parsley, or freshly ground pepper.

❁ Perk Things Up

For a zestier dressing, add a chopped jalapeño pepper (no additional sodium per serving) or 1 tablespoon of a low-sodium fruit salsa, like American Spoon Foods Kiwi Lime Salsa Verde or Mango Habanero Salsa (less than 10 milligrams of sodium per serving). A sweet-peppery option that only adds a trace of sodium to each serving is to stir in 1 teaspoon of American Spoon Foods Jalapeño Jelly.

Layered Fruit and Spinach Salad

Serves 4	
Per serving:	
Calories:	280.97
Protein:	4.91 g
Carbohydrates:	23.88 g
Total fat:	20.03 g
Sat. fat:	1.82 g
Cholesterol:	0.00 mg
Sodium:	210.96 mg
Fiber:	6.17 g

1 large red onion, thinly sliced
1 tablespoon Spectrum Naturals balsamic vinegar
2–3 tablespoons red wine vinegar
2 tablespoons water
1 tablespoon Cascadian Farm frozen Organic Apple Juice Concentrate
2 teaspoons Cascadian Farm frozen Organic Cranberry Juice Concentrate
¼ cup Spectrum Naturals grapeseed oil (or other mild vegetable oil)

1 teaspoon Dijon mustard
¼ teaspoon freshly ground black pepper
¼ cup chopped pecans (and toasted, if desired)
4 cups fresh spinach, cleaned, stemmed, and torn into pieces
1 (5-ounce) can mandarin oranges packed in juice, drained
¼ cup American Spoon Foods dried cranberries

1. Place the red onion slices in a bowl. In a saucepan over medium heat, bring 2 tablespoons of the red wine vinegar, the water, and apple juice concentrate to a boil. Pour the boiling liquid over the onions. Cover and refrigerate, letting the onions "wilt" for at least 1 hour.
2. Combine the balsamic vinegar, cranberry juice concentrate, grapeseed oil, mustard, and pepper in a covered jar. Drain off the liquid from the onions and add it to the jar; set the onions aside. Shake the jar until the mixture is emulsified. Taste and add additional red wine vinegar 1 teaspoon at a time until the desired tartness is achieved.
3. If toasted pecans are preferred, heat a small nonstick sauté pan over medium heat. Add the pecans and toast for 3 minutes, tossing or stirring constantly to prevent them from burning.
4. Place the spinach in a bowl. Shake the jar of salad dressing again (to make sure it's emulsified), pour over the spinach, and toss to coat the spinach. Divide between 4 serving plates.
5. Top each portion with equal parts of the wilted red onion rings, mandarin orange sections, dried cranberries, and pecans. Serve immediately.

Saffron Vinaigrette

Serves 16	
Per serving:	
Calories:	74.24
Protein:	0.03 g
Carbohydrates:	1.65 g
Total fat:	6.75 g
Sat. fat:	0.91 g
Cholesterol:	0.00 mg
Sodium:	0.99 mg
Fiber:	0.00 g

1 cup dry white wine
1 cup rice wine or white wine
  vinegar
1 tablespoon chopped shallot
3 peppercorns, crushed

½ teaspoon dried thyme
¼ teaspoon saffron
½ cup extra-virgin olive oil
½ tablespoon honey

Add the wine, vinegar, shallot, peppercorns, thyme, and saffron to a saucepan over medium-low heat; slowly reduce by half to yield ½ cup of liquid. Strain the mixture through a fine-mesh sieve. Whisk in the olive oil and honey. Use immediately to wilt lettuce, or chill until ready to serve.

Pear Salad with Fat-Free Raspberry Vinaigrette

Serves 4	
Per serving:	
Calories:	420.79
Protein:	5.34 g
Carbohydrates:	21.77 g
Total fat:	36.41 g
Sat. fat:	6.79 g
Cholesterol:	10.71 mg
Sodium:	207.48 mg
Fiber:	3.27 g

2 tablespoons Cascadian Farm
  frozen Organic Raspberry Juice
  Concentrate
2 tablespoons water
1 tablespoon white wine vinegar
1 tablespoon plain nonfat yogurt
⅛ teaspoon freshly ground black
  or white pepper

4 cups mixed salad greens (such
  as iceberg lettuce, green leaf
  lettuce, romaine, and radicchio),
  torn into bite-size pieces
2 medium-size Bartlett pears,
  peeled, sliced, and diced
¼ cup chopped walnuts, toasted
2 ounces bleu cheese, crumbled

1. In a small bowl, combine the raspberry juice concentrate, water, white wine vinegar, yogurt, and pepper; whisk well to combine.
2. Toss the salad greens with the vinaigrette. Divide the greens between 4 serving plates. Top with the pears, nuts, and bleu cheese. Serve immediately.

Grilled Steak Salad

Serves 4	
Per serving:	
Calories:	266.49
Protein:	21.74 g
Carbohydrates:	9.18 g
Total fat:	15.86 g
Sat. fat:	4.76 g
Cholesterol:	159.80 mg
Sodium:	415.46 mg
Fiber:	1.84 g

1 (8-ounce) boneless lean sirloin steak, trimmed of all fat
2 tablespoons Hellmann's or Best Foods Real Mayonnaise
¼ cup plain nonfat yogurt
1 tablespoon Cascadian Farm Sweet Pickle Relish
1 tablespoon lemon juice
1 teaspoon champagne or white wine vinegar
½ teaspoon granulated sugar
¼ teaspoon Dijon mustard
⅛ teaspoon mustard powder
1 tablespoon low-salt ketchup
1 large green onion, white and green parts finely sliced
4 cups lettuce or salad greens mix, torn into bite-size pieces
2 large hard-boiled eggs, sliced
2 tomatoes, cut into wedges
1 ounce bleu cheese, crumbled
Freshly ground black pepper

1. In a nonstick grill pan or on an indoor or outdoor grill, cook the steak for about 2 to 3 minutes per side, or to medium doneness.
2. While the steak cooks, prepare the dressing. In a small bowl, whisk together the mayonnaise, yogurt, relish, lemon juice, vinegar, sugar, mustard, mustard powder, ketchup, and onion.
3. Thinly slice the steak against the grain, then cut the slices into bite-size pieces. Add to the mayonnaise mixture and stir to combine.
4. Divide the lettuce between 4 serving plates. Arrange slices from half a boiled egg and half a tomato on each plate. Evenly divide the mayonnaise-steak dressing mixture among the plates, spooning it atop the lettuce. Top each salad with bleu cheese and freshly ground black pepper.

❀ Flavor Swaps

The ketchup in the mayonnaise dressing for Grilled Steak Salad gives it a taste similar to Russian dressing. If you prefer the flavor of Thousand Island dressing, chop the hard-boiled egg and add it to the dressing instead of serving it alongside the salad. For a saltier-tasting dressing, substitute a lower sodium dill relish like that from Cascadian Farm for the sweet relish.

Warm Broccoli and Potato Salad

6 medium-size potatoes, peeled
  and cubed
2 cups broccoli florets
¼ cup fresh orange juice
3 tablespoons white wine or
  champagne vinegar
½ teaspoon dried basil
1 clove garlic, minced
Pinch dried red pepper flakes

1–2 teaspoons dried parsley
⅛ teaspoon mustard powder
¼ teaspoon Dijon mustard
3 tablespoons extra-virgin olive oil
2 large green onions, white and
  green parts thinly sliced
Freshly ground black or white
  pepper, to taste

Serves 8	
Per serving:	
Calories:	169.17
Protein:	3.17 g
Carbohydrates:	28.26 g
Total fat:	5.52 g
Sat. fat:	0.74 g
Cholesterol:	0.00 mg
Sodium:	99.74 mg
Fiber:	2.69 g

1. Preheat oven to lowest temperature.
2. Place the potatoes in a saucepan and cover with cold water. Bring to a boil, cover, and cook for 10 minutes or until fork tender. Remove the potatoes with a slotted spoon. Save the water, keeping the pan on the heat. Transfer the potatoes to a baking sheet and place in the warm oven.
3. Add the broccoli to the reserved water and blanch for 1 minute. Remove the broccoli with a slotted spoon and add to the potatoes in the oven.
4. In a small saucepan over medium-high heat, combine the orange juice, vinegar, basil, garlic, and dried red pepper flakes; bring to a boil. Remove from heat and whisk in the parsley, mustard powder, mustard, and olive oil. Add the onion and stir to mix.
5. Remove the vegetables from the oven and transfer to a serving bowl. Toss with the dressing, making sure all the potatoes and broccoli florets are thoroughly coated. Top with freshly ground white or black pepper. Serve immediately.

Spiced Tuna Salad with Toasted Sesame Seed Vinaigrette

Serves 2	
Per serving:	
Calories:	253.90
Protein:	18.98 g
Carbohydrates:	6.28 g
Total fat:	17.94 g
Sat. fat:	2.30 g
Cholesterol:	31.25 mg
Sodium:	53.94 mg
Fiber:	1.58 g

2 tablespoons freeze-dried shallots
Boiling water
1 teaspoon sesame seeds
1 tablespoon white wine vinegar
1 tablespoon rice vinegar
1 teaspoon mustard powder
Optional: ¼–½ teaspoon Oriental (hot) mustard powder
¾ teaspoon granulated sugar
2 tablespoons sesame oil
¼ teaspoon toasted sesame oil
¼ teaspoon ground coriander
¼ teaspoon ground star anise
¼ teaspoon ground cinnamon
¼ teaspoon ground cloves
⅛ teaspoon ground ginger
1 (6-ounce) can Chicken of the Sea Very Low Sodium Tuna, drained
1 teaspoon canola (or sesame) oil
2 cups prepared salad greens, torn into bite-size pieces
2 large green onions, white and green parts finely sliced
Optional: Candied ginger

1. Put the freeze-dried shallots in a small bowl. Pour enough boiling water over them to cover. Cover the bowl with plastic wrap and set aside for 5 minutes. Drain the shallots and put them in a blender.
2. Toast the sesame seeds in a small skillet over medium heat until light golden brown.
3. Add the vinegars, mustard powders, and sugar to the shallots in the blender; purée for about 2 minutes. While the blender is running, slowly add both sesame oils. Add the sesame seeds and blend for 1 minute.
4. In small nonstick sauté pan over medium heat, warm the coriander, star anise, cinnamon, cloves, and ginger until fragrant. Transfer the heated spices to a bowl.
5. Drain the tuna and mix it with the canola oil. Add the tuna to the sauté pan, adding the heated spices to taste; sauté until coated with the spices and heated through.
6. Toss the salad greens and sliced green onion with the vinaigrette. Divide between 2 plates. Top each lettuce serving with equal amounts of the sautéed tuna. Garnish with finely shaved slices of candied ginger, if desired.

Thousand Island Dressing

½ cup plain nonfat yogurt
2 tablespoons Hellmann's or Best Foods Real Mayonnaise
2 tablespoons low-salt ketchup
1 tablespoon Cascadian Farm Sweet Relish
1 teaspoon lemon juice
1 teaspoon apple cider vinegar
1 tablespoon finely chopped celery
½ teaspoon granulated sugar or ¼ teaspoon honey
¼ teaspoon celery seed
¼ teaspoon onion powder
¼ teaspoon yellow or Dijon mustard
⅛ teaspoon mustard powder
⅛ teaspoon freshly ground black pepper
1 large hard-boiled egg, minced

Serves 16	
Per serving:	
Calories:	31.74
Protein:	1.24 g
Carbohydrates:	2.71 g
Total fat:	1.90 g
Sat. fat:	0.27 g
Cholesterol:	14.41 mg
Sodium:	70.52 mg
Fiber:	0.48 g

Add all ingredients to a jar. Cover and shake well to combine. Refrigerate between uses. Can be stored 3 to 4 days. To serve, shake well to emulsify.

Russian Dressing

½ cup grapeseed or canola oil
¼ cup red wine or balsamic vinegar (or a combination)
¼ cup water
½ teaspoon Dijon mustard
1 teaspoon garlic powder
1 teaspoon onion powder
¼ teaspoon mustard powder
¼ teaspoon freshly ground black pepper
¼ teaspoon granulated sugar
¼ teaspoon dried basil
¼–½ teaspoon salt-free chili powder
¼–½ teaspoon sweet paprika
2 tablespoons Muir Glen No Salt Added Tomato Paste
Pinch dried red pepper flakes
1 tablespoon finely chopped green bell pepper

Serves 18	
Per serving:	
Calories:	61.48
Protein:	0.39 g
Carbohydrates:	1.16 g
Total fat:	6.27 g
Sat. fat:	0.59 g
Cholesterol:	0.00 mg
Sodium:	78.93 mg
Fiber:	0.29 g

Add all the ingredients to a jar. Cover and shake well to combine. Refrigerate between uses. To serve, shake well to emulsify.

Candied Walnut Salad with Pomegranate Vinaigrette

Serves 4	
Per serving:	
Calories:	290.46
Protein:	5.01 g
Carbohydrates:	27.34 g
Total fat:	19.67 g
Sat. fat:	3.67 g
Cholesterol:	5.32 mg
Sodium:	285.13 mg
Fiber:	6.01 g

⅛ cup chopped walnuts
2 tablespoons sherry
1 tablespoon granulated sugar
2 tablespoons extra-virgin olive oil
1 tablespoon balsamic vinegar
1 teaspoon pomegranate concentrated juice or pomegranate
  molasses
⅛ cup water
¼ teaspoon Dijon mustard
Pinch mustard powder

Pinch freshly ground black pepper
4 cups mixed salad greens, torn
  into bite-size pieces
1 mango or peach, peeled, pitted,
  and diced
1 ripe pear, peeled, cored, and
  diced
1 ripe avocado, peeled, pitted,
  and sliced
1 ounce bleu cheese, crumbled

1. Add the walnuts, sherry, and sugar to a small, nonstick sauté pan over high heat. Stir constantly with a wooden spoon until the sherry and sugar caramelize on the walnuts. Set aside to cool.
2. Add the oil, vinegar, pomegranate juice (or molasses), water, mustard, mustard powder, and pepper to a jar and shake until smooth and creamy.
3. Toss the salad greens, mango (or peach), and pear with the dressing. Divide between 4 serving plates. Arrange the avocado slices evenly around the salads. Top with the crumbled bleu cheese and candied walnuts.

❀ Instant Fat-Free Salad Dressing

Mix some of your favorite fruit jelly with an equal amount American Spoon Foods jalapeño jelly (see Appendix B). Add freeze-dried green onion or shallots and vinegar to taste; thin with a little water, if necessary.

Creamed Chicken Dressing

2 tablespoons nonfat dry milk
¼ teaspoon Minor's Low Sodium
    Chicken Base
½ cup water
½ cup apple cider vinegar
1 large egg
1 tablespoon unbleached
    all-purpose flour
⅛ cup granulated sugar

⅓ teaspoon mustard powder
¼ teaspoon freshly ground black
    pepper
¼ cup Hellmann's or Best Foods
    Real Mayonnaise
¼ cup plain nonfat yogurt
½ teaspoon celery seed
1 cup chopped cooked chicken
    breast, cold

Serves 4	
Per serving:	
Calories:	227.23
Protein:	14.39 g
Carbohydrates:	12.39 g
Total fat:	13.54 g
Sat. fat:	1.98 g
Cholesterol:	91.73 mg
Sodium:	179.13 mg
Fiber:	0.05 g

1. Add the nonfat dry milk, chicken base, water, vinegar, egg, flour, sugar, mustard powder, and pepper to a blender or food processor; pulse to combine.

2. Pour the mixture into a heavy saucepan or top of a double boiler. Cook over medium heat, stirring constantly, until thickened. (To better remove the taste of the raw flour, bring the mixture to a boil, then immediately reduce the heat, whisking the mixture constantly to prevent scorching.) Allow the mixture to cool to room temperature, or refrigerate for a few hours or overnight.

3. Whisk the mayonnaise, yogurt, and celery seed into the cooked dressing. Add the chicken and stir to combine. Serve at room temperature or chilled over salad greens. Top with paprika, if desired.

❖ Quick and Easy Garlic Croutons

Toast four 1-ounce slices of low-salt bread. Use Spectrum Naturals Extra Virgin Olive Spray Oil with Garlic Flavor to spray both sides of the bread. Stack the toast and use a serrated knife to trim off the crusts. Using the same knife, cut the bread into cubes. Place on a baking sheet and set in a 200° oven for 15 minutes or until dried and crispy. Nutritional analysis per serving: Calories: 83.07; Protein: 2.55 g; Carbohydrates: 15.42 g; Total Fat: 1.13 g; Sat. Fat: 0.25 g; Cholesterol: 0.28 mg; Sodium: 8.51 mg; Fiber: 0.00 g.

Waldorf Salad

Serves 4	
Per serving:	
Calories:	287.12
Protein:	4.59 g
Carbohydrates:	24.21 g
Total fat:	21.06 g
Sat. fat:	2.18 g
Cholesterol:	8.40 mg
Sodium:	141.70 mg
Fiber:	4.90 g

1 cup peeled and diced apples
1 tablespoon lemon juice
1 cup diced celery
4 carrots, peeled and finely shredded
½ cup chopped walnuts

¼ cup raisins
¼ cup Hellmann's or Best Foods Real Mayonnaise
¼ cup plain nonfat yogurt
Optional: 4 lettuce leaves

In a bowl, toss the apples with the lemon juice. Add the celery, carrots, walnuts, raisins, mayonnaise, and yogurt; mix well. To serve, place a lettuce leaf on each plate. Evenly divide the salad, scooping it on top of the lettuce leaves.

Tabouleh Salad

Serves 4	
Per serving:	
Calories:	166.33
Protein:	6.58 g
Carbohydrates:	37.67 g
Total fat:	0.96 g
Sat. fat:	0.10 g
Cholesterol:	0.00 mg
Sodium:	60.43 mg
Fiber:	9.41 g

1 cup Now Foods bulgur cracked-wheat cereal, cooked
2 cups boiling water
½ cup chopped fresh parsley
2 large tomatoes, peeled and finely chopped
1 large cucumber, peeled, seeded, and finely chopped

2 carrots, peeled and shredded
2 large stalks celery, diced
2 tablespoons lemon juice
¼ teaspoon freshly ground black pepper
$\frac{1}{16}$–$\frac{1}{8}$ teaspoon mustard powder
1 clove garlic, minced
¼ teaspoon celery seeds

1. Add the bulgur to a large mixing bowl and pour the boiling water over it. Cover and set aside for 30 minutes.
2. Add the remaining ingredients to the bowl and stir to combine. Cover and chill for at least 2 hours. (This gives the salad time to soak in its own juices and brings out the flavor of all the ingredients.)

Italian Dressing

½ cup extra-virgin olive oil
4 cloves garlic, crushed
¼ cup red or white wine vinegar,
   balsamic vinegar, or lemon juice
¼ cup water
¼ teaspoon Dijon mustard
¼ teaspoon mustard powder
¼ teaspoon ground black pepper

¼ teaspoon granulated sugar
½ teaspoon dried basil
¼ teaspoon dried oregano
⅛ teaspoon dried rosemary
⅛ teaspoon dried thyme
Pinch dried red pepper flakes

Serves 16	
Per serving:	
Calories:	65.12
Protein:	0.20 g
Carbohydrates:	0.84 g
Total fat:	6.88 g
Sat. fat:	0.92 g
Cholesterol:	0.00 mg
Sodium:	43.92 mg
Fiber:	0.14 g

Add all the ingredients to a jar. Cover and shake well to combine. Refrigerate overnight to allow the flavors to intensify and combine. Use a slotted spoon to remove and discard the garlic. Refrigerate between uses. To serve, allow 10 minutes for the dressing to come to room temperature and for the olive oil to become liquid again. Shake well to emulsify.

❀ Consider Your Tastes

Always take your own tastes into consideration. If you know you normally don't like spicy dishes, don't cover an entire entrée in a sauce without tasting it first. You may decide you only want to use half the sauce called for in the recipe, or you may want to add additional water or fruit juice to the sauce to mellow the flavor.

Caesar Salad

Serves 4	
Per serving:	
Calories:	213.55
Protein:	7.80 g
Carbohydrates:	20.70 g
Total fat:	11.31 g
Sat. fat:	2.53 g
Cholesterol:	59.60 mg
Sodium:	177.79 mg
Fiber:	1.25 g

4 teaspoons extra-virgin olive oil
1 clove garlic, coarsely chopped
1½ teaspoons Lea & Perrins
  Worcestershire Sauce
1 large egg
2 tablespoons lemon juice
1 tablespoon Hellmann's or Best
  Foods Real Mayonnaise
3 tablespoons plain nonfat yogurt

¼ teaspoon mustard powder
¼ teaspoon ground black pepper
1 tablespoon low-salt ketchup
6 cups mixed salad greens, torn
  into bite-size pieces
1 cup Quick and Easy Garlic
  Croutons (page 53)
4 tablespoons grated Parmesan
  cheese

1. In a small nonstick sauté pan over medium heat, sauté the olive oil and garlic until the oil is warmed, being careful not to brown the garlic (which would impart a bitter flavor). Remove from heat and set aside to allow the garlic flavor to infuse in the oil.
2. In a small bowl, whisk together the Worcestershire sauce, egg, lemon juice, mayonnaise, yogurt, mustard powder, and pepper.
3. Use a slotted spoon to remove and discard the garlic from the olive oil. Return the sauté pan to the burner. Warm the oil over medium heat, then add the egg mixture. Stirring or whisking constantly, heat the mixture until it becomes a thickened sauce. (The lemon juice helps prevent the egg from curdling from the direct heat.) Add the ketchup and whisk to combine. Set aside to cool to room temperature.
4. Toss the salad greens with the dressing. Add the croutons and cheese and toss again. Top with additional freshly ground black pepper.

Crab Louis

¼ cup Hellmann's or Best Foods Real Mayonnaise

¼ cup plain nonfat yogurt

¼ cup French dressing

1 teaspoon tarragon vinegar

¼ teaspoon granulated sugar

1 tablespoon Muir Glen Sweet Relish

1 tablespoon low-salt ketchup

1 tablespoon chopped black olives

1 teaspoon freeze-dried chives (or 1 tablespoon snipped fresh chives)

½ teaspoon horseradish

½ teaspoon Lea & Perrins Worcestershire Sauce

¼ teaspoon freshly ground black pepper

4 cups mixed salad greens

2 cups cooked crabmeat, chilled

4 hard-boiled eggs, finely chopped

Optional: Fresh chives, snipped, for garnish

Optional: Roasted red pepper, cut into strips or chopped, for garnish (see instructions for roasting peppers on page 58)

Serves 4	
Per serving:	
Calories:	293.55
Protein:	13.64 g
Carbohydrates:	7.58 g
Total fat:	23.14 g
Sat. fat:	3.74 g
Cholesterol:	236.95 mg
Sodium:	543.61 mg
Fiber:	1.08 g

1. In a small bowl, mix together the mayonnaise, yogurt, French dressing, vinegar, sugar, relish, ketchup, black olives, chives, horseradish, Worcestershire sauce, and black pepper. (Optional: Mix 1 of the chopped eggs into the dressing.)

2. Toss the salad greens with half of the dressing. Arrange a cup of dressed salad greens on each of 4 plates. Top each salad with the crabmeat, shaped into a mound in the center of the salad. Circle each mound of crabmeat with chopped egg. Make an indentation in the crabmeat and fill with equal portions of the remaining dressing. Garnish with fresh snipped chives, roasted red pepper, and additional freshly ground black pepper, if desired.

Roasted Red (or Other) Peppers

THE TRADITIONAL METHOD of roasting a red pepper is to use a long-handled fork to hold the pepper over the open flame of a gas burner until it's charred. Of course, there are a variety of other methods as well.

- Place the pepper on a rack set over an electric burner and turn it occasionally, until the skin is blackened. This should take about 4 to 6 minutes.
- You can also put the pepper over direct heat on a preheated grill. Use tongs to turn the pepper occasionally.
- Another method is to broil the pepper on a broiler rack about 2" from the heat, turning the pepper every 5 minutes. Total broiling time will be about 15 to 20 minutes, or until the skins are blistered and charred.
- You can also roast a pepper by placing it on a baking sheet treated with nonstick spray and baking it in a 400° oven for 20 to 30 minutes. (The skin of the pepper will not get as dark using this method.)

The key to peeling the peppers is letting them sit in their steam in a closed container until they are cool. Seal the peppers in either a brown paper bag, a plastic bag, or a bowl covered with plastic wrap. Once the peppers are cool, the skin will rub or peel off easily. Keep the pepper whole to peel it, then cut off the top and discard the seeds and rib membrane.

Store roasted peppers in a plastic bag in the refrigerator for a few days. To preserve them for a week, cover the roasted pepper completely with extra-virgin olive oil and refrigerate in an airtight container. Be sure to account for any oil that remains on the roasted pepper when you use it. You can use the oil, too! It absorbs some of the pepper's flavor, and is a delicious addition to salad dressings. ∾

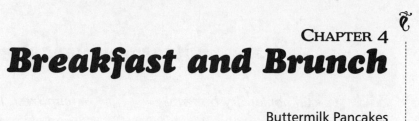

CHAPTER 4

Breakfast and Brunch

Buttermilk Pancakes

Serves 4	
Per serving:	
Calories:	217.32
Protein:	8.54 g
Carbohydrates:	27.87 g
Total fat:	7.62 g
Sat. fat:	1.43 g
Cholesterol:	109.45 mg
Sodium:	463.70 mg
Fiber:	0.84 g

⅛ cup nonfat dry buttermilk
  powder
1 cup unbleached all-purpose flour
2 large eggs, lightly beaten
1 teaspoon granulated sugar
4 teaspoons grapeseed or
  canola oil

⅛ cup fresh lemon juice
½ cup skim milk
¾ cup carbonated water
Spectrum Naturals Grapeseed
  Spray Oil

1. In a small mixing bowl, or in a blender or food processor, mix together the buttermilk powder, flour, eggs, sugar, oil, lemon juice, and skim milk. Immediately prior to making the pancakes, add the carbonated water and fold it into the batter.
2. To prepare the pancakes, pour the batter by spoonfuls or ladle it onto a hot griddle or nonstick skillet treated with the nonstick spray oil. Spread the batter to make thin, crepelike pancakes. Cook over medium heat until the batter bubbles on top. Flip the pancakes and cook for an additional 15 to 30 seconds, until cooked through. Serve immediately with your choice of toppings.

❀ Fruity Matters

It's true that the flavor of freshly squeezed fruit juice is wonderful, but it's not always practical. An (almost) equally delicious alternative is to keep your freezer stocked with fruit juice concentrates and mix your own "fresh" fruit juice as needed. Most lemonade concentrates have sugar added; however, you can get 100% frozen lemon juice from Minute Maid.

Maple Turkey Sausage

Serves 4	
Per serving:	
Calories:	182.96
Protein:	19.90 g
Carbohydrates:	3.36 g
Total fat:	9.43 g
Sat. fat:	2.57 g
Cholesterol:	90.06 mg
Sodium:	107.61 mg
Fiber:	0.00 g

1 pound lean ground turkey
1 tablespoon maple syrup
¼ teaspoon freshly ground black pepper
⅛ teaspoon mustard powder
⅛ teaspoon ground cloves
⅛ teaspoon ground sage
Pinch ground cinnamon
Pinch ground allspice
Pinch ground mace
Optional: ¼ teaspoon natural maple flavoring

1. Mix together all the ingredients in a bowl. Cover and refrigerate overnight.
2. Shape the mixture into 4 flat patties. Cook over medium heat in a nonstick skillet or grill pan for 3 minutes on each side or until cooked through.

Apple-Potato Pancakes

Serves 4	
Per serving:	
Calories:	219.70
Protein:	8.97 g
Carbohydrates:	23.82 g
Total fat:	10.45 g
Sat. fat:	2.02 g
Cholesterol:	212.50 mg
Sodium:	98.02 mg
Fiber:	2.24 g

½ cup Maple Leaf Potato Granules
1½ cups boiling water
4 eggs
2 teaspoons granulated sugar
½ teaspoon ground cinnamon
1 cup peeled and grated Granny Smith or Yellow Delicious apple
¼ cup chopped pecans
Optional: Plain nonfat yogurt, sour cream, or applesauce

1. To prepare the potatoes, add potato granules to a medium-sized bowl. Gradually pour the boiling water over the potato granules, whisking continuously to mix and whip.
2. In a small bowl, beat together the eggs, sugar, and cinnamon. Beat into the potatoes. Fold in the grated apple and chopped pecans.
3. Bring a nonstick skillet or griddle treated with nonstick spray to temperature over medium heat. (If using an electric griddle, preheat to 350° to 380°.) Cook the pancakes on both sides until golden brown. Serve hot—plain or topped with plain nonfat yogurt, sour cream, or applesauce.

Cream and Sugar Breakfast Tarts

Serves 12	
Per serving:	
Calories:	268.82
Protein:	5.51 g
Carbohydrates:	44.33 g
Total fat:	7.63 g
Sat. fat:	3.49 g
Cholesterol:	15.59 mg
Sodium:	236.89 mg
Fiber:	1.23 g

1 recipe Basic White Bread dough (page 212)
Zest of 1 lemon, grated or ⅓ teaspoon minced dehydrated lemon peel
¾ cup plain nonfat yogurt
6 ounces cream cheese, at room temperature
¾ cup powdered sugar
½ teaspoon vanilla extract or ¼–½ teaspoon lemon extract
¼ cup granulated sugar

1. Preheat oven to 450°.
2. Remove the dough from the refrigerator and punch it down. Either in the bowl or on a prepared surface, knead the lemon zest into the bread dough. (If using minced dehydrated lemon peel, first process it into a coarse powder using a mortar and pestle or spice grinder.)
3. Divide the dough into 12 equal segments and work each segment into a ball; set aside to rest for a few minutes.
4. In a bowl, mix together the yogurt, cream cheese, powdered sugar, and vanilla (or lemon) extract until smooth.
5. Flatten or roll out each dough segment into 6" rounds. Carefully transfer the dough to a baking sheet treated with nonstick spray. Press down the center of each round, leaving an unpressed border around each piece. Use a fork to poke holes in the centers. (This helps prevent the tarts from rising too high in the center during baking, which would cause the cream cheese topping to run off.) Evenly divide the cream cheese mixture between the rounds, spreading it onto the centers of the dough rounds. Sprinkle 1 teaspoon of granulated sugar over the top of each filled dough round.
6. Bake until the tarts are puffed and golden brown, about 20 to 25 minutes. Remove from the oven and let sit for about 3 minutes (so the cream and sugar solidifies and the tarts are easier to handle). Serve warm. Sprinkle with a dusting of powdered sugar over the top, if desired.

Sausage and Egg Casserole

1 (16-ounce) bag Cascadian Farm
  Country Style Potatoes
Spectrum Naturals Olive Oil or
  Super Canola Spray Oil
8 eggs
4 teaspoons Hellmann's or Best
  Foods Real Mayonnaise
¼ teaspoon garlic powder
¼ teaspoon onion powder
¼ teaspoon freshly ground black
  pepper

¼ teaspoon mustard powder
1 cup skim milk
8 (1-ounce) slices Bread Machine
  Potato Water Sourdough Oat
  Bran Bread (page 222)
¼ pound Peppery Turkey Sausage
  (page 68), cooked and crumbled
½ cup shredded Swiss cheese
4 tablespoons grated Parmesan
  cheese

Serves 8	
Per serving:	
Calories:	261.01
Protein:	16.22 g
Carbohydrates:	25.81 g
Total fat:	10.78 g
Sat. fat:	4.04 g
Cholesterol:	234.51 mg
Sodium:	318.42 mg
Fiber:	2.32 g

1. Preheat oven to 350°. Spray an 11" × 7" × 1½" oven-safe casserole
   dish with the spray oil.
2. Add the frozen potatoes to a microwave-safe bowl; cover and microwave
   at 50 percent power for 3 to 5 minutes, until thawed and warm.
3. In a large mixing bowl, beat the eggs with the mayonnaise, garlic
   powder, onion powder, pepper, mustard powder, and milk. Tear the
   bread into bite-size pieces and stir them into the egg mixture. Fold the
   thawed potato mixture, the sausage, and grated Swiss cheese into the
   egg mixture. Pour into the prepared casserole dish. Sprinkle the grated
   Parmesan cheese evenly over the top of the casserole.
4. Bake for approximately 35 to 45 minutes, until the eggs are set, the
   cheese is bubbling, and the top of the casserole is golden brown.
   Let sit for 5 minutes, then slice and serve.

❋ Zapping Sausage

*You can prepare the sausage for the Sausage and Egg Casserole by
precooking it in the microwave. Put the sausage in a microwave-safe
dish; cover, and microwave at 70 percent power for 3 to 5 minutes,
turning the bowl halfway through the cooking time. Drain off the fat.
Break the sausage apart with a fork.*

Veggie Pancakes

Serves 8	
Per serving:	
Calories:	83.58
Protein:	3.67 g
Carbohydrates:	11.03 g
Total fat:	2.86 g
Sat. fat:	0.98 g
Cholesterol:	29.18 mg
Sodium:	207.86 mg
Fiber:	1.38 g

4 large carrots, peeled and grated
1 cup seeded and grated zucchini
1 large sweet onion, finely chopped
1 stalk celery, finely chopped
½ cup unbleached all-purpose flour
½ teaspoon low-salt baking powder
⅛ teaspoon mustard powder

1/16 teaspoon salt
¼ teaspoon pepper
1 egg
¼ cup skim milk
2 teaspoons canola oil
Spectrum Naturals Super Canola Spray Oil or other nonstick spray

1. Add the carrots, zucchini, onion, and celery to a microwave-safe bowl. Cover and microwave on high for 4 minutes or until the vegetables are tender and the onion is transparent. Set aside to cool.

2. In a small bowl, thoroughly combine the flour, baking powder, mustard powder, salt, and pepper. In a larger bowl, beat together the egg, milk, and oil. Add the dry ingredients and stir until combined. Fold in the carrots, zucchini, and onion.

3. Bring a large nonstick skillet or griddle treated with nonstick spray to temperature over medium heat. Make a few pancakes at a time by ladling about ¼ cup of batter per pancake onto the heated pan surface. Cook for about 2 minutes on each side. Serve immediately.

❁ Keeping Pancakes Warm
Cooked pancakes can be transferred to a baking sheet and placed in a warm oven (150° to 200°) to be kept warm while you prepare the rest of the pancakes and remaining meal entrées.

Country Breakfast Strata

1 teaspoon olive oil

1 teaspoon unsalted butter

½ pound Peppery Turkey Sausage
   (page 68)

⅛ teaspoon dried sage

1 small sweet onion, chopped

1 red bell pepper, seeded and
   chopped

1 green bell pepper, seeded and
   chopped

8 large eggs

½ teaspoon mustard powder

1 cup skim milk

½ cup shredded Cheddar cheese

6 (1-ounce) slices low-salt bread,
   cut into ½" cubes

Optional: Tomato slices

Optional: Fresh basil and parsley

Serves 8	
Per serving:	
Calories:	434.19
Protein:	29.82 g
Carbohydrates:	25.11 g
Total fat:	23.09 g
Sat. fat:	8.47 g
Cholesterol:	487.88 mg
Sodium:	279.70 mg
Fiber:	1.39 g

1. Heat the oil and butter in a sauté pan on medium; sauté the sausage for 2 minutes. Add the sage and mix with the sausage. Add the onion and peppers; sauté until the onion is transparent.

2. In a large mixing bowl, beat together the eggs and mustard powder. Whisk in the skim milk. Stir in the sausage mixture, Cheddar cheese, and bread cubes. Transfer to an oven-safe 11" × 7" casserole dish treated with nonstick spray. Cover and refrigerate overnight.

3. Remove the casserole dish from refrigerator. Preheat oven to 350°. Bake the strata, uncovered, for 45 minutes or until the eggs are set. Let rest for 5 minutes, then cut into 8 pieces. Serve with slices of fresh tomato and garnished with basil and parsley, if desired.

❖ Italian-Seasoned Strata

Convert the Country Breakfast Strata to a dish with an Italian influence by substituting ½ teaspoon of Mrs. Dash Classic Italiano Seasoning Blend for the sage and 1 ounce each of shredded Swiss cheese and grated Parmesan cheese for the Cheddar. Nutritional analysis per serving: Calories: 436.23; Protein: 31.26 g; Carbohydrates: 25.44 g; Total Fat: 22.48 g; Sat. Fat: 8.10 g; Cholesterol: 485.17 mg; Sodium: 342.38 mg; Fiber: 1.39 g.

Garlic-Roasted Potatoes Frittata

Serves 4	
Per serving:	
Calories:	224.12
Protein:	15.60 g
Carbohydrates:	34.20 g
Total fat:	3.10 g
Sat. fat:	1.20 g
Cholesterol:	4.00 mg
Sodium:	246.66 mg
Fiber:	0.39 g

9 small red potatoes, thinly sliced
Spectrum Naturals Extra Virgin
   Olive Spray Oil with Garlic
   Flavor
2 teaspoons olive oil
1 cup thinly sliced leeks
1 cup thinly sliced zucchini
1 clove garlic, minced
2 teaspoons dried basil

1 teaspoon balsamic vinegar
¼ teaspoon mustard powder
1½ cups frozen egg substitute,
   thawed
¼ cup grated Parmesan cheese
¼ teaspoon freshly ground black
   pepper

1. Preheat oven to 400°. Treat a baking sheet with the spray oil.
2. Arrange the potatoes in a single layer on the prepared baking sheet. Spray the tops of the potatoes with a thin coating of the spray oil. Bake for 15 minutes or until tender.
3. Bring the oil to temperature over medium-high heat in a large, deep, oven-safe nonstick sauté pan. Add the leeks and zucchini; sauté for 2 minutes. Lower the temperature and add the garlic; sauté until the leeks and zucchini are tender, stirring to avoid burning the garlic. Add the basil, vinegar, and mustard powder; stir to combine. Spread out the mixture evenly across the bottom of the pan. Add the roasted potatoes in an even layer to the pan.
4. Mix the egg substitute with half of the grated Parmesan cheese and pour over the vegetables in the pan. Tilt the pan to ensure the egg substitute goes to the edges of the pan. Use a spatula to move the vegetables to ensure they're all coated with the egg substitute. Cook until almost set. Sprinkle the top of the frittata with the pepper and remaining Parmesan cheese.
5. Bake for 5 to 10 minutes, or until the cheese is melted and the top of the frittata is lightly browned. Use a spatula to loosen the frittata from the pan and slide it out onto a serving plate. Slice and serve.

Breakfast Pudding

2 small zucchini, grated
1 small sweet onion, minced
1 clove garlic, minced
3 cups no-salt-added sweet corn
   (if fresh, cut from about 6 ears
   of corn)
6 carrots, peeled and shredded
1 cup evaporated skim milk,
   divided
1 tablespoon unbleached all-purpose flour
1½ tablespoons cornmeal

1 cup (1% fat) cottage cheese
2 eggs
½ teaspoon dried thyme
¼ teaspoon mustard powder
¼ teaspoon freshly ground black
   pepper
⅛ teaspoon dried lime granules,
   crushed
Spectrum Naturals Canola Spray
   Oil with Butter Flavor
1 tablespoon bread crumbs

Serves 4	
Per serving:	
Calories:	282.32
Protein:	20.70 g
Carbohydrates:	42.60 g
Total fat:	5.10 g
Sat. fat:	1.50 g
Cholesterol:	115.17 mg
Sodium:	381.66 mg
Fiber:	2.85 g

1. Preheat oven to 325°.
2. Add the zucchini, onion, garlic, corn, and carrots to a microwave-safe casserole dish. Cover and microwave on high for 3 minutes; turn bowl and microwave on high for an additional 3 minutes. Leave the cover in place and set aside.
3. Whisk together ½ cup of the milk, the flour, and cornmeal in a microwave-safe bowl; microwave on high for 1 minute. Whisk again and continue to microwave in 30-second increments, whisking between each time, until the mixture has thickened.
4. Combine the remaining ½ cup milk, the cottage cheese, eggs, thyme, mustard powder, pepper, and lime granules in a blender or food processor; process until smooth and well-mixed. Add the cottage cheese mixture to the corn mixture; stir to combine.
5. Treat an 11" × 7" oven-safe casserole dish with the spray oil. Transfer the corn mixture to the casserole dish. Spread the cornmeal mixture over the top of the corn mixture. Sprinkle the bread crumbs over the top. Spray lightly with the spray oil. Bake for 1 hour. Let stand for 5 minutes. Serve hot.

Peppery Turkey Sausage

Serves 8	
Per serving:	
Calories:	84.93
Protein:	9.95 g
Carbohydrates:	0.00 g
Total fat:	4.71 g
Sat. fat:	1.28 g
Cholesterol:	45.03 mg
Sodium:	53.58 mg
Fiber:	0.00 g

1 pound lean ground turkey
¼ teaspoon garlic powder
¼ teaspoon onion powder
¼ teaspoon dried sage

½ teaspoon freshly ground black pepper
⅛ teaspoon ground cloves
Pinch ground allspice

1. In a mixing bowl, combine all the ingredients until well-mixed. Form into 8 equal-sized patties.
2. Pan-fry in a nonstick grill pan or prepare in a covered indoor grill (such as a George Foreman—style indoor grill). The sausage is done when the juices run clear.

Strawberry Egg White Pancakes

Serves 4	
Per serving:	
Calories:	93.59
Protein:	8.23 g
Carbohydrates:	13.85 g
Total fat:	0.33 g
Sat. fat:	0.06 g
Cholesterol:	0.00 mg
Sodium:	112.62 mg
Fiber:	0.71 g

½ cup oatmeal
8 egg whites
1 tablespoon lemon juice

2 tablespoons strawberry jam
⅛ cup unbleached all-purpose flour

1. Process the oatmeal in a blender or food processor until ground. Whisk the egg whites in a metal or glass bowl until soft peaks form. Mix the lemon juice and jam together (to thin the jam and make it easier to fold into the egg whites). Fold the thinned jam, ground oatmeal, and flour into the egg whites.
2. Preheat a nonstick pan or griddle treated with cooking spray over medium heat. Pour one-fourth of the mixture into the pan and cook for about 4 minutes or until the top of pancake bubbles and begins to get dry. Flip the pancake; cook until the inside of the cake is cooked. Repeat until the remaining 3 pancakes are done.

Cheddar-Cheesy Sausage Muffins

1 large Granny Smith apple,
  peeled, cored, and grated
1 tablespoon lemon juice
½ cup plain nonfat yogurt
½ pound Peppery Turkey Sausage,
  cooked, drained, and crumbled
  (page 68)

2 teaspoons honey
⅛ teaspoon ground cinnamon
¼ cup shredded Cheddar cheese
4 Thomas' English muffins, split
Spectrum Naturals Canola Spray
  Oil with Butter Flavor

Serves 4	
Per serving:	
Calories:	324.04
Protein:	18.42 g
Carbohydrates:	44.99 g
Total fat:	8.15 g
Sat. fat:	3.53 g
Cholesterol:	52.98 mg
Sodium:	329.96 mg
Fiber:	1.45 g

1. Preheat oven to 350°.
2. Toss the grated apple with the lemon juice; set aside.
3. Place the yogurt between several layers of paper towels for 10 to 15 minutes. Place the grated apple between layers of paper towels and blot dry. Use a spatula to scrape the yogurt and apple into a bowl. Add the cooked sausage, honey, cinnamon, and Cheddar cheese; mix well.
4. Lightly spray the tops and bottoms of the muffins with the spray oil. Place each of the bottom sections of the muffins on a piece of non-stick aluminum foil. Evenly divide the Cheddar mixture between the 4 muffin halves. Place the muffin tops over the coated bottom halves. Wrap the muffins in the foil. Bake for 20 minutes or until heated through and the cheese is melted.

✿ Make Sandwiches Instead!

If you prefer, rather than bake the Cheddar-Cheesy Sausage Muffins, you can make open-face sandwiches by first toasting the muffins, then spraying the tops and bottoms with the spray oil. Place the muffin halves (sprayed-sides down) on a baking sheet and top with the Cheddar mixture. Place under the broiler until the cheese is melted and bubbly.

Buckwheat Pancakes

Serves 4	
Per serving:	
Calories:	234.03
Protein:	10.27 g
Carbohydrates:	44.65 g
Total fat:	2.32 g
Sat. fat:	0.67 g
Cholesterol:	54.96 mg
Sodium:	70.78 mg
Fiber:	3.81 g

½ cup whole-wheat flour
½ cup unbleached all-purpose flour
½ cup buckwheat flour
1½ teaspoons low-salt baking powder
1 large egg
3 tablespoons Cascadian Farm frozen Organic Apple Juice Concentrate
1 tablespoon lemon juice
1¼–1½ cups skim milk

1. Sift the flours and baking powder together. Combine the egg, apple juice concentrate, lemon juice, and 1¼ cups of the skim milk. Add the milk mixture to the dry ingredients and mix well, but do not overmix. Add the remaining milk if necessary to reach desired consistency. (This will be according to how you like your pancakes.)
2. Cook the pancakes in a nonstick skillet or on a griddle treated with nonstick spray over medium heat. The pancakes are ready to turn over after bubbles appear on the surface.

Overnight Fruit and Oatmeal

Serves 4	
Per serving:	
Calories:	226.18
Protein:	8.33 g
Carbohydrates:	41.53 g
Total fat:	3.94 g
Sat. fat:	1.19 g
Cholesterol:	4.27 mg
Sodium:	18.02 mg
Fiber:	6.00 g

1 cup steel-cut oats
14 dried apricot halves
1 dried fig
2 tablespoons golden raisins
4 cups water
½ cup whole milk
¼ teaspoon cinnamon
⅛ teaspoon dried orange granules, crushed
Pinch ground cloves
Pinch ground ginger
Pinch ground allspice

Combine all the ingredients in a slow-cooker with a ceramic interior; set to low heat. Cover and cook overnight (for 8 to 9 hours).

Fruit Smoothie

½ cup frozen strawberries,
  unsweetened
1 tablespoon Cascadian Farm
  frozen Organic Apple Juice
  Concentrate

3 tablespoons water
½ medium-size banana, sliced
8 ounces peach nonfat yogurt

Put all the ingredients in a blender or food processor and process
until thick and smooth.

Serves 2	
Per serving:	
Calories:	135.18
Protein:	4.46 g
Carbohydrates:	32.94 g
Total fat:	0.18 g
Sat. fat:	0.06 g
Cholesterol:	0.00 mg
Sodium:	72.92 mg
Fiber:	1.49 g

Tofu Smoothie

1 cup frozen unsweetened peach
  slices
1 large banana, sliced
½ cup soft silken tofu

2 teaspoons honey
4 teaspoons toasted wheat germ
Chilled water, as needed

Put all the ingredients in a food processor or blender and process
until smooth. Add a little chilled water, if necessary.

Serves 2	
Per serving:	
Calories:	168.82
Protein:	5.15 g
Carbohydrates:	35.26 g
Total fat:	2.40 g
Sat. fat:	0.42 g
Cholesterol:	0.00 mg
Sodium:	4.37 mg
Fiber:	4.04 g

Apple-Spiced Egg Clouds on Toast

Serves 2	
Per serving:	
Calories:	208.78
Protein:	9.34 g
Carbohydrates:	32.47 g
Total fat:	5.12 g
Sat. fat:	2.65 g
Cholesterol:	10.62 mg
Sodium:	117.51 mg
Fiber:	3.46 g

4 egg whites
1 teaspoon powdered sugar, sifted
2 teaspoons unsalted butter
1 large apple, peeled, cored, and
  thinly sliced
2 teaspoons lemon juice
1 teaspoon brown sugar

¼ teaspoon cinnamon
Pinch ground cloves
Pinch ground ginger
Pinch ground allspice
2 cups water
2 slices low-salt bread
Optional: Freshly ground nutmeg

1. In a metal or glass bowl, beat the egg whites until they thicken. Add the powdered sugar, and continue to beat until stiff peaks form.
2. Heat a small sauté pan on medium; add the butter. Toss the apple slices in the lemon juice and add them to the pan. Sprinkle the brown sugar, cinnamon, cloves, ginger, and allspice over the apples; sauté, stirring occasionally, until the apples are tender and glazed.
3. While the apples cook, bring the water to a simmer in a large, deep nonstick sauté pan over medium-low heat. Drop the egg whites by the tablespoonful into the simmering water. Simmer for 3 minutes, then turn the egg white "clouds" over and simmer for an additional 3 minutes.
4. Toast the bread and divide the apples over the slices, then top with the "clouds." Sprinkle with nutmeg, if desired. Serve immediately.

❉ Egg-citing News

While 1 egg has 6 grams of high-quality protein, the good news is that it also has 25 percent of the daily requirement of vitamin B_{12} and moderate amounts of folic acid and minerals. Don't be fooled by the high cholesterol content of eggs either. Research has shown that eating foods containing saturated fat is far more likely to raise a person's blood cholesterol level than eating foods containing cholesterol. In fact, egg yolk is high in lecithin, a cholesterol-lowering agent, and is a source of pantothenic acid, a vitamin that aids in sodium metabolism.

Lemon Crepes

2 large eggs
¾ cup unbleached all-purpose flour
1 tablespoon lemon juice
⅛ teaspoon lemon extract
1 cup skim milk

1 tablespoon nonfat dry milk
⅛ teaspoon low-salt baking
    powder
Pinch baking soda

Serves 10	
Per serving:	
Calories:	59.56
Protein:	3.21 g
Carbohydrates:	8.85 g
Total fat:	1.14 g
Sat. fat:	0.36 g
Cholesterol:	43.07 mg
Sodium:	48.68 mg
Fiber:	0.26 g

1. Combine all the ingredients in a blender or food processor and process until the mixture is the consistency of cream.
2. Treat an 8" nonstick skillet with nonstick spray and heat on medium. Pour about 2 tablespoons of the crepe batter into the hot pan, tilting in a circular motion until the batter spreads evenly over the pan. Cook the crepe until the outer edges just begin to brown and loosen. Flip the crepe to the other side and cook for about 30 seconds. Using a thin spatula, slide the crepe from the pan onto a warm plate or baking sheet set in a warm oven. Continue until all the crepes are done.
3. Serve by placing fresh fruit or a little jelly in a line in the center of the crepe. Roll the crepe and place seam-side down on the plate. Dust with a little powdered sugar or Whey Low powder (see Appendix B) for a more attractive presentation.

❀ Lemon Yields

On average, a medium-sized lemon will yield ⅛ cup (2 tablespoons) of juice and 2 teaspoons of lemon zest. Like herbs, the ratio for fresh to dry lemon zest is a third; in other words, if a recipe calls for 1 teaspoon of fresh lemon zest, you can substitute ⅓ teaspoon of dried lemon granules or dried lemon peel. (The same ⅓ rule applies to dried versus fresh lime or orange zest as well.)

CHAPTER 5
Chicken Entrées

Crunchy Oven-Fried Chicken Thighs

Serves 4	
Per serving:	
Calories:	100.67
Protein:	9.54 g
Carbohydrates:	6.41 g
Total fat:	3.87 g
Sat. fat:	0.71 g
Cholesterol:	34.03 mg
Sodium:	226.25 mg
Fiber:	0.19 g

4 chicken thighs, skin removed
1 tablespoon unbleached all-purpose flour
1 large egg white
¼ teaspoon sea salt
½ teaspoon olive oil
1 tablespoon rice flour
1 tablespoon cornflakes crumbs
Nonstick cooking spray

1. Preheat oven to 350°.
2. Rinse and dry the chicken thighs. Put the flour on a plate. In a small, shallow bowl, whip the egg white together with the sea salt; add the olive oil and mix it into the egg white. Put the rice flour and cornflakes crumbs on another plate and mix them together.
3. Roll each chicken thigh in the flour, then dip it into the egg white mixture, and then roll it in the cornflakes crumbs mixture. Place a rack on a baking sheet and spray with the nonstick cooking spray. Arrange the chicken thighs on the rack so that they aren't touching. Bake for 35 to 45 minutes, until the meat juices run clear. (Note: If not using a rack, drain the thighs on paper towels to remove the excess fat before serving.)

❁ Sack the Sodium
You can reduce the sodium in Crunchy Oven-Fried Chicken Thighs to 85.31 mg per serving by omitting the salt and substituting a herb blend like Mrs. Dash Table Blend, the Spice House's Mr. Spice House Salt-Free Blend, or the Spice Hunter All Purpose Chef's Blend.

Cajun-Style Chicken

4 (4-ounce) boneless, skinless
   chicken breasts
2 teaspoons olive oil
½ teaspoon paprika
½ teaspoon cayenne pepper
¼ teaspoon onion powder
¼ teaspoon garlic powder
¼ teaspoon freshly ground black
   pepper

¼ teaspoon freshly ground white
   pepper
⅛ teaspoon dried oregano
⅛ teaspoon dried thyme
⅛ teaspoon dried basil
⅛ teaspoon dried rosemary
Optional: ¼ teaspoon brown sugar

Serves 4	
Per serving:	
Calories:	149.00
Protein:	26.40 g
Carbohydrates:	0.90 g
Total fat:	3.80 g
Sat. fat:	0.70 g
Cholesterol:	66.00 mg
Sodium:	74.00 mg
Fiber:	0.20 g

1. Put the chicken breasts and olive oil in a heavy-duty, sealable plastic bag. Turn the bag to completely coat the chicken in the oil.
2. In a bowl, mix together the remaining ingredients. Dip the top half of each chicken breast in the dried seasoning mixture.
3. Heat a nonstick skillet or grill pan on medium-high. Place the chicken breasts in the skillet, spice-coated side down. Cook for 2 to 3 minutes or until the top half of the chicken begins to lose its pinkish color and the spiced side of the chicken is browned well, almost blackened. Use tongs to turn the chicken. Cook for 1 minute or until the chicken is done.

❧ Quicker Seasoning Mixes

Don't be afraid to do some experimenting and come up with your own "personalized" salt-free seasoning blends. You don't have to start from scratch to do so. For example, for Cajun-Style Chicken, try mixing a blend such as ½ teaspoon each of Mrs. Dash Garlic and Herb, Classic Italiano, Minced Onion Medley or Onion and Herb, and Extra Spicy Seasoning Blends.

Grilled Chicken Breast with Mustard Sauce

Serves 4	
Per serving:	
Calories:	181.98
Protein:	27.03 g
Carbohydrates:	2.93 g
Total fat:	6.13 g
Sat. fat:	1.92 g
Cholesterol:	71.03 mg
Sodium:	261.49 mg
Fiber:	0.51 g

4 (4-ounce) boneless, skinless chicken breasts
¼ teaspoon freshly ground black pepper
2 teaspoons olive oil
2 teaspoons unsalted butter
⅛ cup minced shallots or red onion
⅛ teaspoon ground brown mustard seeds, crushed
¼ teaspoon mustard powder

Pinch dried rosemary
Pinch dried thyme
Pinch dried sage
1 tablespoon white wine or dry white vermouth
1 teaspoon malt vinegar
¼ teaspoon Minor's Low Sodium Chicken Base
1 teaspoon cornstarch
½ cup water
¼ teaspoon Dijon mustard

1. Preheat a George Foreman–style indoor grill. Season the chicken with the freshly ground black pepper. Grill for 3 to 4 minutes, until the chicken is cooked through and the juices run clear.
2. In a nonstick sauté pan, heat the olive oil over medium heat. Add the butter. When the butter sizzles, add the shallots (or onion); sauté until tender. Add the ground brown mustard seeds, mustard powder, rosemary, thyme, and sage; stir well.
3. Add the white wine (or vermouth) and vinegar; stir well, and cook for 1 minute. Add the Minor's base and stir to blend with the mixture in the pan.
4. Add the cornstarch to the water and mix well, whisking to remove any lumps. Add to the pan and bring to a boil. Reduce heat and simmer until thickened.
5. Remove pan from heat and whisk in the Dijon mustard. Pour over the grilled chicken breasts. Serve immediately.

Steamed Chili-Peppered Chicken

¼ teaspoon ground ancho pepper
¼ teaspoon ground chipotle
  pepper
⅛ teaspoon dried marjoram
Pinch ground cumin
¼ teaspoon dried Mexican oregano

⅛ teaspoon dried thyme
⅛ teaspoon ground cloves
1 teaspoon garlic powder
1 tablespoon white wine vinegar
4 boneless, skinless chicken thighs

Serves 4	
Per serving:	
Calories:	135.47
Protein:	22.28 g
Carbohydrates:	0.22 g
Total fat:	4.43 g
Sat. fat:	1.13 g
Cholesterol:	94.12 mg
Sodium:	97.56 mg
Fiber:	0.00 g

1. In a small bowl, mix together the ancho pepper, chipotle pepper, marjoram, cumin, oregano, thyme, cloves, and garlic powder.
2. In a separate bowl, pour the vinegar over the chicken, turning the chicken to evenly coat it in the vinegar.
3. Cut out four 16" squares of parchment paper. Dip the vinegar-coated chicken in the seasoning mixture, coating both sides. Place each thigh in the center of a parchment-paper square. Bring the 4 corners together and tie closed with string. Place in a steamer and steam over simmering water for 1 hour.

❋ Steaming Tips

If you steam several vegetables at once, cut the denser vegetables that require the longest cooking time into smaller pieces than those vegetables that cook the quickest. If steaming a meat entrée and vegetables, consult the estimated steaming times for both; you may need to add the vegetables to the steamer sometime after you start steaming the entrée. Be sure to add an additional 1 or 2 minutes to the cooking time to compensate for opening the steamer.

Chicken Cacciatore

Serves 4	
Per serving:	
Calories:	217.22
Protein:	27.48 g
Carbohydrates:	12.64 g
Total fat:	5.97 g
Sat. fat:	0.99 g
Cholesterol:	65.77 mg
Sodium:	126.20 mg
Fiber:	2.17 g

4 teaspoons olive oil
1 large sweet onion, diced or sliced
4 (4-ounce) boneless, skinless chicken breasts
¼ teaspoon freshly ground black pepper
2 tablespoons dry red wine
1 (15-ounce) can Muir Glen Organic No Salt Added Tomato Sauce
1 teaspoon garlic powder

½ teaspoon dried basil
¼ teaspoon dried oregano
¼ teaspoon dried parsley
⅛ teaspoon mustard powder
Pinch dried lemon granules, crushed
Pinch dried red pepper flakes
1 teaspoon lemon juice
¼ teaspoon granulated sugar
Optional: 4 tablespoons grated Parmesan cheese

1. Heat a deep nonstick skillet on medium. Add the olive oil and chopped onion; sauté the onion until transparent. Push to the edges of the pan.
2. Add the chicken breasts. Sprinkle the pepper over the chicken. Pan-fry for 2 minutes on each side. Use tongs to transfer the chicken breasts to a bowl or platter; set aside.
3. Add the wine to the pan. Bring to a boil and cook for 2 minutes, stirring the wine into the onion and using the spoon or spatula to scrape (deglaze) the bottom of the pan.
4. Add the tomato sauce, garlic powder, basil, oregano, parsley, mustard powder, lemon granules, red pepper flakes, lemon juice, and sugar to the pan; stir to combine.
5. Add the chicken back to the pan, spooning some of the tomato sauce over the top of the chicken. Reduce heat. Simmer, covered, for 45 minutes. Serve immediately, topped with freshly grated Parmesan cheese.

Red and Green Bell Pepper Chicken

4 teaspoons olive oil

1 green bell pepper, seeded and
   chopped

1 red bell pepper, seeded and
   chopped

2 cloves garlic, minced

4 (4-ounce) boneless, skinless
   chicken thighs

¼ teaspoon freshly ground black
   pepper

2 tablespoons dry red or white wine

1 (14.5-ounce) can Muir Glen
   Organic No Salt Added Diced
   Tomatoes

1 teaspoon dried basil

½ teaspoon dried parsley

⅛ teaspoon dried marjoram or
   oregano

1 teaspoon lemon juice

¼ teaspoon granulated sugar

Serves 4	
Per serving:	
Calories:	209.08
Protein:	23.38 g
Carbohydrates:	6.28 g
Total fat:	8.98 g
Sat. fat:	1.75 g
Cholesterol:	94.12 mg
Sodium:	135.80 mg
Fiber:	1.07 g

1. Heat a deep nonstick skillet on medium. Add the olive oil and
   chopped bell peppers; sauté until tender. Add the garlic and sauté for
   1 minute, being careful not to burn the garlic. Push the mixture to the
   edges of the pan.
2. Add the chicken thighs. Sprinkle the pepper over the chicken. Pan-fry
   for 2 minutes on each side. Use tongs to transfer the chicken to a
   bowl or platter; set aside.
3. Add the wine to the pan. Bring to a boil and cook for 2 minutes, stirring the wine into the peppers and using the spoon or spatula to
   scrape (deglaze) the bottom of the pan.
4. Add the tomatoes, basil, parsley, marjoram (or oregano), lemon juice,
   and sugar to the pan; stir to combine.
5. Add the chicken back to the pan, spooning some of the tomatoes
   over the top of the chicken. Reduce heat. Simmer, covered, for
   35 minutes. Serve immediately.

Olive Oil and Lemon Herbed Chicken

Serves 4	
Per serving:	
Calories:	216.57
Protein:	22.33 g
Carbohydrates:	1.13 g
Total fat:	12.60 g
Sat. fat:	2.91 g
Cholesterol:	94.12 mg
Sodium:	143.01 mg
Fiber:	0.04 g

4 boneless, skinless chicken thighs
4 teaspoons olive oil
⅛ teaspoon dried marjoram or oregano
¼ teaspoon dried parsley
⅛ teaspoon dried rosemary
⅛ teaspoon dried thyme or lemon thyme

¼ teaspoon garlic powder
2 tablespoons dry white wine
½ teaspoon cornstarch
2 tablespoons fresh lemon juice
4 teaspoons Spectrum Naturals Non-Hydrogenated Organic Margarine

1. Add the chicken thighs and olive oil to a heavy-duty, sealable plastic bag. Close the bag and turn it to coat each chicken piece completely.
2. In a small bowl, mix together the marjoram, parsley, rosemary, thyme, and garlic powder.
3. Heat a nonstick skillet on medium-high. Dip the chicken thigh tops in the herb seasoning mixture. Place the chicken in the skillet, herb-coated side down. Add any residual olive oil from the bag to the skillet. Fry the chicken for 2 to 3 minutes on each side or until the juices run clear. Transfer the cooked chicken to a serving platter.
4. Add the wine to the skillet, stirring and scraping the bottom of the pan (deglaze) to remove any chicken "bits." Add any herbs remaining in the bowl to the pan. Bring the wine to a boil.
5. Stir the cornstarch into the lemon juice, whisking to remove any lumps. Add the lemon juice and bring to a boil. Reduce heat, stirring constantly, simmering the mixture until it thickens.
6. Remove the pan from the heat and whisk in the margarine. Pour over the chicken and serve immediately.

❈ Fat Facts

Using a butter-flavored margarine in the Olive Oil and Lemon Herbed Chicken recipe doesn't significantly drop the overall fat content of the recipe; however, it does drop the less healthful saturated fat content. Using unsalted butter, the saturated fat for the recipe would be 4.13 g.

Java Chicken Paprika

1 pound boneless, skinless chicken breasts
½ cup fresh lemon juice
¼ teaspoon freshly ground black pepper
1 tablespoon olive oil
1 large sweet onion, sliced
2 teaspoons paprika

½ teaspoon salt-free chili powder
½ teaspoon instant espresso powder
¼ cup water
1 tablespoon cornstarch
1 tablespoon instant nonfat dry milk
½ cup skim milk
Optional: Additional paprika, for garnish

Serves 4	
Per serving:	
Calories:	200.97
Protein:	28.16 g
Carbohydrates:	10.18 g
Total fat:	4.96 g
Sat. fat:	0.91 g
Cholesterol:	66.58 mg
Sodium:	100.88 mg
Fiber:	0.59 g

1. Place the chicken breasts between pieces of waxed paper or plastic wrap. Pound the breasts into thin pieces using a wooden mallet or rolling pin. Divide into 4 equal-sized pieces.
2. Place the chicken breasts in a small bowl. Pour the lemon juice over the chicken and season with the freshly ground black pepper. Marinate for at least 5 minutes. Drain and pat dry, reserving the lemon juice.
3. In a large nonstick skillet, heat the olive oil on medium. Add the onion and sauté until transparent. Remove the onion with a slotted spoon and set aside.
4. Increase the heat to medium-high. Add the chicken breasts to the pan. Quick-fry the chicken breasts for about 1 minute on each side. Transfer the chicken to a serving platter and keep warm.
5. Add the onion back to the pan and reheat. Add the paprika and chili powder; stir well. Add the espresso powder and water; bring to a boil.
6. Whisk together the cornstarch, nonfat dry milk, and skim milk. Add the milk mixture and the reserved lemon juice to the pan; bring to a boil. Reduce heat and simmer, stirring until thickened.
7. Spoon the sauce over the chicken. Sprinkle with additional paprika, if desired. Serve immediately.

Yogurt "Gravy" Chicken Thighs

Serves 4	
Per serving:	
Calories:	355.01
Protein:	32.20 g
Carbohydrates:	45.60 g
Total fat:	4.70 g
Sat. fat:	1.28 g
Cholesterol:	96.38 mg
Sodium:	214.86 mg
Fiber:	5.64 g

1 (16-ounce) package Cascadian Farm Hash Browns

1 (10-ounce) package Cascadian Farm Gardener's Blend frozen vegetables

1 large sweet onion, sliced

4 (4-ounce) boneless, skinless chicken thighs

¼ teaspoon freshly ground black pepper

1 teaspoon garlic powder

1 tablespoon cornstarch

1 teaspoon dried parsley

2 cups plain nonfat yogurt

1 teaspoon za'atar or herb seasoning blend

1. Preheat oven to 350°.
2. Place the hash browns, frozen vegetables, and onion in an oven- and microwave-safe casserole dish treated with nonstick spray. Cover with plastic wrap and microwave on high for 3 minutes. Turn the dish and microwave on high for an additional 2 to 3 minutes, until the vegetables are thawed and the onion is tender.
3. Remove and discard the plastic wrap. Season the chicken with the pepper and garlic powder. Arrange the thighs over the top of the vegetable mixture.
4. Stir the cornstarch and parsley into the yogurt. Pour the mixture over the chicken and vegetable mixture, spreading the yogurt so that it covers everything in an equal layer.
5. Bake for 45 minutes or until the yogurt is bubbling and thickened and the chicken thighs are done. Sprinkle the thighs with the za'atar. Serve immediately.

❀ Za'atar's the Star
Za'atar is a mixture of sumac, sesame seeds, and herbs like oregano and hyssop. It's often used in Middle Eastern dishes.

Herbed Chicken Paprikash

4 (8-ounce) chicken leg quarters, skin removed
Spectrum Naturals Extra Virgin Olive Spray Oil with Garlic Flavor
¼ teaspoon dried marjoram or oregano
¼ teaspoon dried thyme
¼ teaspoon dried basil
⅛ teaspoon dried rosemary
⅓ cup dry white wine
⅓ cup low-sodium chicken broth
⅔ cup fresh button mushrooms, sliced
¼ cup finely grated carrots
2 tablespoons unbleached all-purpose flour
2 tablespoons water
1 teaspoon paprika
2 tablespoons plain nonfat yogurt
Additional paprika, for garnish

Serves 4	
Per serving:	
Calories:	203.00
Protein:	28.90 g
Carbohydrates:	5.70 g
Total fat:	6.20 g
Sat. fat:	1.50 g
Cholesterol:	108.00 mg
Sodium:	133.00 mg
Fiber:	0.50 g

1. Bring a deep nonstick skillet to temperature over medium heat. Spray both sides of the chicken with the nonstick spray. Sprinkle the chicken with the marjoram (or oregano), thyme, basil, and rosemary. Add the chicken to the skillet and cook for 2 minutes on each side or until browned.
2. Add the wine and chicken broth to pan; bring to a boil. Reduce heat, cover, and simmer for 20 minutes. Add the mushrooms and carrots, cover, and simmer for an additional 10 minutes. Use tongs to transfer the chicken to a serving plate. Keep warm.
3. Mix together the flour and water, whisking to remove any lumps. Add the mixture to the pan and increase heat to medium; bring to a boil, stirring constantly. Continue to cook over medium heat, stirring until the mixture thickens.
4. Stir in the paprika. Remove from heat and stir in the yogurt. Pour the sauce over the chicken. Sprinkle with additional paprika, if desired.

* Nutritional analysis for 1-ounce boneless, skinless chicken breast (white meat):

Serves 4

Per serving:	
Calories:	46.78
Protein:	8.79 g
Carbohydrates:	0.00 g
Total fat:	1.01 g
Sat. fat:	0.29 g
Cholesterol:	24.10 mg
Sodium:	20.98 mg
Fiber:	0.00 g

* Nutritional analysis for 1-ounce boneless, skinless chicken thigh (dark meat):

Per serving:	
Calories:	59.25
Protein:	7.35 g
Carbohydrates:	0.00 g
Total fat:	3.08 g
Sat. fat:	0.86 g
Cholesterol:	26.93 mg
Sodium:	24.95 mg
Fiber:	0.00 g

Seasoned Chicken

Parts of chicken, with skin, either white or dark meat

Seasoning blend of your choice from the following recipes

1. Preheat oven to 375°.
2. Mix together the ingredients from the seasoning blend to make a paste.
3. Wash chicken pieces under cold running water. Pat dry with a paper towel. Carefully pull back the skin, using the tip of a boning knife, if necessary, to loosen the membrane under the skin from the meat. Evenly rub the seasoning paste directly on the meat. Pull the skin back to cover the meat. Place a roasting rack inside a roasting pan and treat with nonstick spray. Arrange the chicken pieces on the rack so that they aren't touching. (Juices that drain from the meat and the baked "bits" that adhere to the roasting pan can be used in sauces or gravy provided you first drain off any fat.)
4. Bake until the juices run clear—about 40 minutes for legs or thighs and about 50 minutes for whole chicken breasts. Reduce baking times by 10 minutes if using boneless, skin-on chicken pieces. Remove from the oven and allow the meat to rest on the rack for 5 to 10 minutes. Pull the skin away from the meat, using a boning knife, if necessary, to cut away the still-attached end. (The skin can usually just be torn off.) Serve immediately.

❀ Poultry Primer

A heart-healthy menu calls for smaller meat entrées. When you plan your meals to include lots of grains, vegetables, and fruit, 3 to 4 ounces is usually a sufficient serving of meat. As a general rule, a whole chicken breast is split in half to yield 2 servings. The cooked-meat yield (minus the bones) will depend on the size of the breast, but is usually around 6 ounces per half breast, so a whole breast is sometimes enough for 4 servings. The cooked-meat yield for a chicken leg will be around 2 ounces; a thigh will yield 3 to 4 ounces, on average.

Seasoning Blends

Fine Herbes Chicken

1 teaspoon lemon juice
¼ teaspoon dried parsley
¼ teaspoon dried chervil
¼ teaspoon dried tarragon
¼ teaspoon freeze-dried chives
¹⁄₁₆ teaspoon dried orange granules, crushed

Spiced Orange Chicken

1 teaspoon Cascadian Farm frozen
Organic Orange Juice Concentrate
¼ teaspoon honey
¼ teaspoon garlic powder
⅛ teaspoon freshly ground black pepper
¹⁄₁₆ teaspoon ground cinnamon
Pinch ground cloves
Pinch ground allspice
Pinch ground mace

Zesty Lemon Herb Chicken

2 teaspoons lemon juice
2 teaspoons freeze-dried shallots
¼ teaspoon marjoram
¼ teaspoon thyme
¼ teaspoon rosemary
⅛ teaspoon salt-free chili powder
2 drops lemon oil

Chili-Jalapeño Chicken

2 teaspoons jalapeño jelly
¼ teaspoon onion powder
¼ teaspoon garlic powder
¼ teaspoon (hot or sweet) paprika
¼ teaspoon chili pepper
⅛ teaspoon oregano
⅛ teaspoon thyme
Pinch ground cumin
Pinch ground coriander
Pinch cayenne
¹⁄₁₆ teaspoon dried lemon granules, crushed

Herbes de Provence Chicken

¼ teaspoon dried basil
¼ teaspoon dried marjoram
¼ teaspoon dried thyme
⅛ teaspoon dried mint
⅛ teaspoon dried rosemary
⅛ teaspoon fennel seeds
⅛ teaspoon dried lavender
¹⁄₁₆ teaspoon dried lemon granules, crushed
1 teaspoon white dry wine
(or enough to form a paste)

Chili-Bourbon Chicken

2 teaspoons bourbon
1 teaspoon Lea & Perrins Worcestershire Sauce
1 teaspoon Muir Glen Organic
No Salt Added Tomato Paste
2 teaspoons freeze-dried green onion
¼ teaspoon garlic powder
⅛ teaspoon freshly ground black pepper
⅛ teaspoon chili powder
Pinch cayenne pepper
Optional: Salt-free hickory smoke or
mesquite base (powder), to taste

Apple-Jalapeño Chicken

1 tablespoon applesauce
1 teaspoon apple cider vinegar
1 tablespoon freeze-dried shallots
1 teaspoon jalapeño jelly
¼ teaspoon garlic powder
⅛ teaspoon freshly ground black pepper
Optional: ⅛ teaspoon chipotle powder
Optional: ¼ teaspoon brown sugar

Jamaican Jerk Roasted Chicken

⅛ teaspoon dried lime granules, crushed
⅛ teaspoon ground ginger
¼ teaspoon onion powder
⅛ teaspoon allspice
¼ teaspoon garlic powder
⅛ teaspoon sweet paprika
⅛ teaspoon dried thyme
⅛ teaspoon freshly ground black pepper
Pinch dried cloves
Pinch cayenne
1 teaspoon jalapeño jelly

Herbed Chicken and Broccoli Casserole

2 cups broccoli
½ pound cooked chicken, chopped
½ cup skim milk
2 tablespoons Hellmann's or Best Foods Real Mayonnaise
1 cup plain nonfat yogurt
½ teaspoon Minor's Low Sodium Chicken Base
¼ cup Maple Leaf Potato Granules (or other unseasoned, no-fat-added instant mashed potato flakes or potato flour)
⅛ teaspoon dried oregano

¼ teaspoon dried parsley
¼ teaspoon garlic powder
¼ teaspoon onion powder
⅛ teaspoon celery seeds
⅛ teaspoon freshly ground black pepper
1 large egg, beaten
1 tablespoon lemon juice
½ cup grated Cheddar cheese
½ cup commercial bread crumbs
Spectrum Naturals Canola Spray Oil with Butter Flavor

Serves 4	
Per serving:	
Calories:	356.79
Protein:	30.76 g
Carbohydrates:	23.41 g
Total fat:	15.78 g
Sat. fat:	5.66 g
Cholesterol:	118.82 mg
Sodium:	331.94 mg
Fiber:	2.91 g

1. Preheat oven to 350°. Treat an 11" × 7" casserole dish with nonstick spray.
2. Steam the broccoli until tender; drain. Spread out the chicken on the bottom of the prepared dish and cover it with the broccoli.
3. Put the milk, mayonnaise, yogurt, chicken base, potato granules, oregano, parsley, garlic powder, onion powder, celery seeds, pepper, egg, and lemon juice in a blender or the bowl of a food processor and pulse until well-mixed; pour over the broccoli. Mix together the cheese and bread crumbs; spread the mixture over the top of the casserole. Lightly spray the top of the crumbs with the butter-flavored spray. Bake for 30 minutes.

Quick Skillet Chicken Casserole

Serves 4	
Per serving:	
Calories:	307.71
Protein:	23.13 g
Carbohydrates:	35.72 g
Total fat:	8.06 g
Sat. fat:	2.03 g
Cholesterol:	47.84 mg
Sodium:	151.25 mg
Fiber:	5.03 g

½ cup skim milk
2 tablespoons Hellmann's or Best Foods Real Mayonnaise
1 cup water
½ teaspoon Minor's Low Sodium Chicken Base
¼ cup Maple Leaf Potato Granules (or other unseasoned, no-fat-added instant mashed potato flakes or potato flour)
½ teaspoon onion powder
¼ teaspoon garlic powder
¼ teaspoon dried celery flakes
⅛ teaspoon freshly ground black pepper
1 large egg, beaten
1 teaspoon Lea & Perrins Worcestershire Sauce
1 tablespoon lemon juice
1 (10-ounce) package Cascadian Farm Gardener's Blend frozen vegetables, thawed
1 cup sliced button mushrooms
½ pound cooked chicken, chopped
1⅓ cups cooked brown, long-grain rice

1. Add the milk, mayonnaise, water, chicken base, potato granules, onion powder, garlic powder, celery flakes, pepper, egg, Worcestershire sauce, and lemon juice to a blender or the bowl of a food processor; pulse until well mixed.
2. Pour the mixture into a large, deep nonstick sauté pan; bring to a boil. Reduce heat and simmer, stirring until the mixture begins to thicken.
3. Add the frozen vegetables, mushrooms, and chicken; stir to combine. Cover and simmer for 5 minutes or until the mushrooms are cooked. Serve over the rice.

❀ Sensible Seasoning

Lemon juice, dried lemon granules, and mustard powder are used often in the recipes in this book. They enhance the flavor in a way similar to salt without increasing the sodium content of the dish. Likewise, the commonly seen ingredient of "salt to taste" has been omitted from the recipes. The reasons for that are obvious; however, if you feel you must add salt to something before you cook it, only add a pinch.

Yogurt "Fried" Chicken

Spectrum Naturals Extra Virgin
    Olive Spray Oil with Garlic
    Flavor
4 (1-ounce) slices French Bread
    (page 216)
1 pound boneless, skinless chicken
    breasts (trimmed of fat)
1 teaspoon garlic powder

1 teaspoon paprika
¼ teaspoon mustard powder
¼ teaspoon dried thyme
2 teaspoons Citrus Pepper (page
    278)
1 cup nonfat plain yogurt

Serves 4	
Per serving:	
Calories:	279.97
Protein:	38.41 g
Carbohydrates:	20.40 g
Total fat:	3.76 g
Sat. fat:	1.06 g
Cholesterol:	88.45 mg
Sodium:	139.85 mg
Fiber:	0.65 g

1. Preheat oven to 350°. Treat a baking pan with the spray oil.
2. Place the bread in the bowl of a food processor or in a blender; process to make bread crumbs.
3. Cut the chicken breasts into 8 equal-sized strips. In a medium-size bowl, combine the garlic powder, paprika, mustard powder, thyme, and Citrus Pepper with the yogurt and mix well. Add the chicken to the yogurt mixture, stirring to make sure all sides of the strips are covered. Lift the chicken strips out of the yogurt mixture and dredge all sides in the bread crumbs. Lightly mist the breaded chicken pieces with the spray oil and arrange in the pan.
4. Bake for 10 minutes. Use a spatula or tongs to turn the chicken pieces. Optional: For the last 5 minutes of cooking, place the pan under the broiler to give the chicken a deep golden color. Watch closely to ensure the chicken "crust" doesn't burn.

❉ Garlic Yields

Each head of garlic usually has 10 to 15 cloves. As a rule, 1 minced clove of garlic will yield ½ teaspoon. When substituting garlic powder, use ⅛ teaspoon of powder (not garlic salt) for each clove of garlic, or vice versa.

Indoor-Grilled Chicken Breast

Serves 4	
Per serving:	
Calories:	194.89
Protein:	30.77 g
Carbohydrates:	3.12 g
Total fat:	5.62 g
Sat. fat:	1.36 g
Cholesterol:	85.05 mg
Sodium:	58.45 mg
Fiber:	0.00 g

1 teaspoon cider vinegar
1 teaspoon garlic powder
4 teaspoons Mr. Spice Honey
   Mustard Sauce
1 teaspoon brown sugar

1 teaspoon Citrus Pepper (page 278)
2 teaspoons olive oil
4 (4-ounce) boneless, skinless
   chicken breast cutlets

1. In a medium-size bowl, combine the cider vinegar, garlic powder, mustard sauce, brown sugar, and Citrus Pepper. Slowly whisk in the olive oil to thoroughly combine and make a paste.
2. Rinse the chicken cutlets and dry between paper towels. If necessary to ensure a uniform thickness of the cutlets, put them between sheets of plastic wrap or wax paper and pound to flatten them.
3. Pour the marinade into a heavy-duty (freezer-style) sealable plastic bag. Add the chicken cutlets, moving them around in the mixture to coat all sides. Seal the bag, carefully squeezing out as much air as possible. Refrigerate and allow the chicken to marinate for at least 1 hour, or as long as overnight.
4. Preheat an indoor (George Foreman–style) grill. When the grill is heated, place the chicken on the grill. Close the grill lid and cook the cutlets for 3 minutes or until the juices run clean.

❁ Go Natural!

Most processed foods have high sodium levels that result from the combination of salt added to the food and the high sodium content of the preservatives. Deciding to do all you can to keep the foods you eat as close to natural as possible is a healthy goal.

Chicken Curry

4 teaspoons olive or canola oil

4 (4-ounce) boneless, skinless
   chicken breast fillets

1 large Vidalia onion, chopped

2 teaspoons Curry Powder (see
   page 263)

¼ teaspoon freshly ground black
   pepper

⅛ cup unbleached all-purpose flour

⅛ cup unsweetened, no-salt-added
   applesauce

1 cup skim milk

Serves 4	
Per serving:	
Calories:	224.09
Protein:	29.47 g
Carbohydrates:	11.23 g
Total fat:	6.17 g
Sat. fat:	1.10 g
Cholesterol:	67.00 mg
Sodium:	111.27 mg
Fiber:	0.65 g

1. Bring a large, deep nonstick sauté pan to temperature over medium heat. Add the oil.
2. Rinse the chicken breasts under cold water, then pat dry between paper towels. Add the chicken to the pan and sauté for 2 minutes on each side. Remove from the pan and keep warm.
3. Add the onion and sauté until transparent. Add the curry powder and pepper; mix with the onion. Stir in the flour and applesauce to create a roux. Increase the heat to medium-high. Gradually whisk in the milk, and bring to a boil. Reduce heat to medium-low to maintain a simmer. Add the chicken back to the pan. Cover and simmer for 5 minutes or until the chicken is cooked through and the "gravy" is thickened.

❈ Microwave Sautéing Instructions

If you're watching your fat, you can omit the oil in most recipes that call for sautéed aromatic vegetables (onion, shallots, celery, etc.) by cooking the vegetables in the microwave instead of sautéing them on the stove. Put the vegetables in a covered microwave-safe bowl. Microwave on high until the onion is transparent and all the vegetables are tender. It usually isn't necessary to add liquid because there is usually enough moisture in the vegetables; however, if you prefer, you can add 1 tablespoon of water or broth—or a mixture of mostly water or broth and a teaspoon of oil for a reduced-fat alternative— to help ensure the vegetables don't dry out.

Quick Indoor-Grilled Chicken Breast

Serves 4	
Per serving:	
Calories:	157.86
Protein:	26.39 g
Carbohydrates:	4.16 g
Total fat:	3.04 g
Sat. fat:	0.86 g
Cholesterol:	72.29 mg
Sodium:	63.10 mg
Fiber:	0.01 g

*4 (4-ounce) frozen boneless, skin-
less chicken breasts*
*1 teaspoon Cascadian Farm frozen
Organic Apple Juice Concentrate*

*4 tablespoons Mr. Spice Honey
Mustard Sauce*
1 teaspoon lemon juice
1 teaspoon Citrus Pepper (page 278)

1. Plug in indoor grill. Rinse the frozen chicken breasts under cold water
   and place immediately on the grill. Close the lid. Grill for 5 to 6 minutes or until the juices run clear.
2. While the chicken grills, add the remaining ingredients to a small
   microwave-safe bowl. Immediately before serving, microwave on high
   for 30 seconds to heat the sauce. Evenly divide over the grilled
   chicken breasts and serve immediately.

Grilled Jerk Chicken

Serves 4	
Per serving:	
Calories:	142.81
Protein:	26.54 g
Carbohydrates:	1.87 g
Total fat:	2.55 g
Sat. fat:	0.53 g
Cholesterol:	65.77 mg
Sodium:	129.95 mg
Fiber:	0.21 g

*1 teaspoon Jerk Spice Blend
(page 278)*
1 teaspoon Bragg Liquid Aminos
2 teaspoons fresh lime juice
1 teaspoon olive or canola oil
1 jalapeño, seeded and chopped

*2 scallions, white and green part
chopped*
1 teaspoon granulated sugar
Pinch mustard powder
*4 (4-ounce) boneless, skinless
chicken breasts*

1. Preheat a George Foreman–style indoor grill.
2. Add all the ingredients *except* the chicken to a small food processor
   or blender and purée.
3. Rinse the chicken in cold water and pat dry between paper towels. Rub
   both sides with the spice mixture. Grill for 3 to 4 minutes, until the
   chicken is cooked through and the juices run clear. Serve immediately.

Seafood Entrées

Sesame Snapper

Serves 4	
Per serving:	
Calories:	163.52
Protein:	24.97 g
Carbohydrates:	2.64 g
Total fat:	5.39 g
Sat. fat:	0.87 g
Cholesterol:	42.42 mg
Sodium:	103.84 mg
Fiber:	0.54 g

1 tablespoon nonfat yogurt
1 teaspoon Hellmann's or Best Foods Real Mayonnaise
1 teaspoon olive or canola oil
1/4 cup unseasoned bread crumbs
2 tablespoons white sesame seeds
1/4 teaspoon coarsely ground white or black pepper
1/8 teaspoon dried lemon peel
1/8 teaspoon dried orange peel
1/8 teaspoon garlic powder
1/8 teaspoon onion powder
4 (4-ounce) snapper fillets
Nonstick spray

1. Preheat oven to 350°.
2. In a shallow bowl, combine the yogurt, mayonnaise, and oil.
3. In another shallow bowl, combine the bread crumbs with the sesame seeds. Measure the pepper, lemon and orange peel, and garlic and onion powders into spice grinder or use a mortar and pestle to "crunch" the dried peel and mix and release the flavors of the dried seasoning. Add to the bread crumb blend and mix well.
4. Rinse the fillets in cold water and pat dry. Brush the skinless side of each fillet with the yogurt blend and then press into the bread crumb mixture.
5. Treat a large, nonstick, oven-safe skillet with nonstick spray. Bring the skillet up to temperature over moderate heat. (Be careful not to get the skillet too hot or the sesame seeds will burn.) Add the fillets to the pan, crumb-side down, and sauté until golden brown. Turn the fillets and sauté until cooked through.
6. If the fillets are large, finish cooking them in the oven until cooked through.

Baked Orange Roughy in White Wine

4 (4-ounce) orange roughy fillets
2 tablespoons dry white wine
1 tablespoon lemon juice
1 teaspoon dried basil

½ teaspoon lemon zest
Optional: Freshly ground white or
    black pepper

Serves 4	
Per serving:	
Calories:	84.40
Protein:	16.69 g
Carbohydrates:	0.47 g
Total fat:	0.79 g
Sat. fat:	0.02 g
Cholesterol:	22.67 mg
Sodium:	71.84 mg
Fiber:	0.07 g

1. Preheat oven to 425°. Treat a baking dish with nonstick spray.
2. Rinse the fish fillets in cold water and pat dry. Pour the wine and lemon juice into the prepared dish. Arrange the fillets in the dish, tucking under thin ends if necessary so the fillets are in an even layer. Sprinkle the basil and lemon zest evenly over the fish. Season with pepper, if desired.
3. Cover the dish with foil. Bake until opaque through the thickest part, about 12 to 18 minutes, depending on the thickness of the fillets. Serve immediately.

Orange-Steamed Fish

4 (4-ounce) orange roughy or
    other mild fish fillets
½ cup sliced celery
¼ cup orange juice
⅛ teaspoon onion powder

⅛ teaspoon garlic powder
⅛ teaspoon black pepper
Pinch each of dried basil, mustard
    powder, oregano, and thyme
4 thin orange slices

Serves 4	
Per serving:	
Calories:	93.17
Protein:	17.00 g
Carbohydrates:	3.52 g
Total fat:	0.88 g
Sat. fat:	0.03 g
Cholesterol:	22.67 mg
Sodium:	85.04 mg
Fiber:	0.58 g

1. Rinse the fish fillets in cold water and pat dry with paper towels. Arrange the sliced celery on the steaming tray of a steamer or on steaming insert for a traditional stovetop pan. Place the fish fillets on top of the celery. Mix the orange juice with the seasonings and spoon evenly over the fish. Top with the orange slices.
2. Set the steaming tray over the boiling water and cover tightly with the lid. Steam the fish until it is opaque through to the center of the thickest part, about 6 to 10 minutes, depending on the thickness of the fillets and the steaming method. Serve immediately.

Stovetop-Poached Halibut with Herbed Lemon Sauce

Serves 4	
Per serving:	
Calories:	131.02
Protein:	24.00 g
Carbohydrates:	3.04 g
Total fat:	2.70 g
Sat. fat:	0.38 g
Cholesterol:	34.85 mg
Sodium:	62.15 mg
Fiber:	1.41 g

4 (4-ounce) halibut fillets
1 lemon
$\frac{1}{3}$ cup mixture fresh herb sprigs
 (parsley, dill, chives, and/or
 chervil) and/or celery leaves

$\frac{1}{4}$ teaspoon black peppercorns
1 bay leaf

1. Rinse the fish fillets in cold water and pat dry.
2. Put 2 to 3 inches of water in a pan broad enough to hold the fillets without overlapping them.
3. Cut the lemon in half. Squeeze the juice from 1 half and reserve for later. Thinly slice the remaining half lemon, reserving 2 slices to cut in half for garnish.
4. Add the lemon slices, herbs, peppercorns, and bay leaf to the water and bring to a boil. Reduce the heat and add the fillets; simmer until the fish is opaque through the thickest part (cut to test), or for about 8 to 10 minutes for fillets that are 1" thick. Transfer the fish to a plate and cover with foil to keep warm.
5. Strain and discard all but 1 cup of the poaching liquid. Bring the reserved poaching liquid to a boil over high heat until it is reduced by half, about 1 to 2 minutes. Stir in the reserved lemon juice. Arrange the halibut on 4 plates and spoon the lemon herb sauce over the fish. Serve immediately garnished with the reserved lemon slices.

❋ Kiss a Fish

Fish is the ultimate convenience food, as it cooks to perfection easily and quickly. It can be baked, broiled, grilled, or steamed in minutes, and when combined with a fresh salad or steamed vegetables, it makes a nutritious, heart-healthy meal. Fish contains high amounts of omega-3 fatty acids, which lower blood pressure and improve blood circulation. Adding fish to your menus will save meal preparation time and satisfy a wide variety of appetites.

Microwave-Poached Salmon

4 (4-ounce) center-cut salmon fillets
1 tablespoon white wine or 1 teaspoon frozen white grape juice
  concentrate mixed with 2 teaspoons water

3 tablespoons water
½ teaspoon Mrs. Dash Lemon
  Pepper
⅛ teaspoon fennel seeds

Serves 4	
Per serving:	
Calories:	212.56
Protein:	22.57 g
Carbohydrates:	0.10 g
Total fat:	12.30 g
Sat. fat:	2.47 g
Cholesterol:	66.87 mg
Sodium:	67.46 mg
Fiber:	0.00 g

1. Place the salmon fillets in a deep, microwave-safe casserole dish. Add the wine (or grape juice mixture) and water. Evenly divide the lemon pepper and fennel seeds over the fillets.
2. Cover and microwave on high for 6 minutes or until the fish just turns opaque throughout and flakes easily when tested with a fork. Serve immediately.

Pan-Seared Flounder Fillets

4 teaspoons olive oil
4 (4-ounce) flounder fillets

1–2 teaspoons Cajun Spice Blend
(page 274)

Serves 4	
Per serving:	
Calories:	191.65
Protein:	21.64 g
Carbohydrates:	0.00 g
Total fat:	11.14 g
Sat. fat:	1.63 g
Cholesterol:	68.00 mg
Sodium:	57.80 mg
Fiber:	0.00 g

1. In a cast-iron frying pan, heat the olive oil until smoking. Coat both sides of the flounder with the Cajun seasoning. Place the coated flounder in the pan and cook for 2 to 3 minutes per side (depending on thickness) until cooked through.
2. Serving suggestion: Transfer the flounder to a serving dish and place on top of mixed greens. Spoon Pomegranate Pizzazz Salsa (page 255) or other favorite salsa or fruit vinaigrette on top of the fish. If you prefer the flavor of a milder condiment to mellow the Cajun spices used on the fish, serve with some fruit, chutney, or a dollop of plain nonfat yogurt and lemon juice.

Shrimp with Chive Butter Sauce

Serves 4	
Per serving:	
Calories:	158.81
Protein:	23.15 g
Carbohydrates:	2.13 g
Total fat:	5.86 g
Sat. fat:	2.79 g
Cholesterol:	182.71 mg
Sodium:	180.02 mg
Fiber:	0.02 g

1 pound cooked shrimp
½ cup water
¼ teaspoon Minor's Low Sodium Chicken Base
1 teaspoon cornstarch
1–2 tablespoons cold water
1 tablespoon lemon juice
¼ cup chopped fresh chives
¼ teaspoon freshly ground white pepper
4 teaspoons cold unsalted butter
Optional: 1 drop lemon oil or ⅛ teaspoon dried lemon granules

1. Bring the water to a boil in a saucepan. Add the chicken base and stir to mix. Combine the cornstarch and cold water to make a slurry, whisking to remove any lumps. Whisk the slurry into the broth. Bring the mixture to a boil again, then reduce the heat. Simmer, whisking constantly until the mixture thickens.
2. Remove from heat. Add the lemon juice and whisk to combine. Stir in the chives and pepper. (If you prefer a more intense lemon flavor, add the optional lemon oil or lemon granules at this time.) Add the cold butter, 1 teaspoon at a time, whisking to combine with the sauce. Serve over shrimp immediately.

❀ Lemon-Seasoned Bread Crumbs

Mildly flavored fish, such as catfish, cod, halibut, orange roughy, rockfish, and snapper, benefit from the distinctive flavor of lemon. Lemon also reduces the need for salt. Adding slices of lemon to the top of the fish infuses the fillets with the citrus flavor. Grated lemon or lime zest is a great way to enhance that flavor or give a flavor boost to a crunchy bread crumb topping for fish.

Orange Roughy with Italian Roasted Vegetables

Spectrum Naturals Extra Virgin
  Olive Spray Oil
¾ pound orange roughy or other
  mild, firm white fish
1 (10-ounce) package Cascadian
  Farm Gardener's Blend frozen
  vegetables
1 (14.5-ounce) can Muir Glen
  Organic No Salt Added Diced
  Tomatoes

1 teaspoon roasted garlic powder
½ teaspoon dried minced onion
½ teaspoon dried basil
¼ teaspoon dried parsley
⅛ teaspoon dried oregano
⅛ teaspoon granulated sugar
1 tablespoon grated Parmesan
  cheese

Serves 4	
Per serving:	
Calories:	138.13
Protein:	18.52 g
Carbohydrates:	13.33 g
Total fat:	0.77 g
Sat. fat:	0.02 g
Cholesterol:	22.10 mg
Sodium:	135.37 mg
Fiber:	3.33 g

1. Preheat oven to 375°. Treat a 2- to 3-quart baking pan or casserole dish with the nonstick spray.
2. Rinse the fish with cold water and pat dry.
3. Place the frozen vegetable blend in an even layer across the bottom of the prepared pan. Place the fish atop the vegetables. Pour the tomatoes and juices evenly over the top. Spray a thin layer of the nonstick spray over the top of the tomatoes.
4. Sprinkle the garlic powder, minced onion, basil, parsley, oregano, and sugar over the top of the tomatoes.
5. Cover the baking pan with aluminum foil or a lid and bake for 45 minutes. Remove the cover (being careful not to burn yourself on the steam). Sprinkle the cheese over the top of the dish. Bake for an additional 15 to 20 minutes or until the cheese is melted and the fish is opaque.

❋ Salt-Free Blend Substitute

Sunny Singapore seasoning is a salt-free blend available from the Spice House (see Appendix B) that combines the flavors of curry spices, lemon, and a blend of white and black pepper and other spices.

Paella

Serves 6	
Per serving:	
Calories:	413.11
Protein:	47.32 g
Carbohydrates:	27.50 g
Total fat:	11.55 g
Sat. fat:	2.58 g
Cholesterol:	191.52 mg
Sodium:	288.91 mg
Fiber:	1.71 g

1 cup uncooked long-grain brown rice
4 teaspoons olive oil
¼ pound boneless, skinless chicken breast
¼ pound boneless, skinless chicken thighs
¼ pound pork tenderloin
½ teaspoon freshly ground black pepper
⅛ teaspoon ground cloves
Pinch dried pepper flakes
1 large sweet onion, diced
4 cloves garlic, minced

1 large green bell pepper, seeded and diced
1 large red bell pepper, seeded and diced
2 stalks celery, diced
2 cups water
1½ teaspoons Minor's Low Sodium Chicken Base
¼ teaspoon Minor's Ham Base
Pinch saffron
1 pound cod
1 pound medium-size shrimp, peeled and deveined

1. Cook rice to al dente according to package directions.
2. Cut the chicken and tenderloin into 1" pieces. Heat the olive oil in a large pan on medium-high. Add the meat to the oil. Season the meat with the pepper, cloves, and pepper flakes; sauté for 3 minutes or until the meat is about medium-rare. Add the onion, garlic, peppers, and celery; sauté until the onion is transparent. Add the rice and sauté for several minutes, stirring it into the meat and onion mixture.
3. Add the water, the bases, and saffron; bring to a boil. Cover, reduce heat, and let simmer for 15 minutes.
4. Rinse the cod in cold water. Cut into 1" cubes and add to the paella. Cover and simmer for 10 minutes. Rinse the shrimp under cold water and add to the paella. Simmer, uncovered, until the shrimp turns pink, about 5 minutes.

Triple Ginger Stir-Fried Scallops and Vegetables

1 pound scallops

1 teaspoon peanut or sesame oil

1 tablespoon chopped fresh ginger

1 tablespoon freeze-dried shallots

1/4 teaspoon freshly ground China Number One Ginger

1 teaspoon minced candied ginger

1 teaspoon rice wine vinegar

2 teaspoons Bragg Liquid Aminos

1/4 teaspoon Minor's Low Sodium Chicken Base

1/2 cup water

2 (10-ounce) packages Cascadian Farm frozen Organic Chinese Stirfry Vegetables

Optional: 4 scallions, thinly sliced

1 teaspoon cornstarch

1–2 tablespoons cold water

1/4 teaspoon toasted sesame oil

Serves 4	
Per serving:	
Calories:	157.27
Protein:	23.00 g
Carbohydrates:	15.03 g
Total fat:	1.41 g
Sat. fat:	0.19 g
Cholesterol:	37.48 mg
Sodium:	329.85 mg
Fiber:	3.40 g

1. Rinse the scallops and pat dry between layers of paper towels. If necessary, slice the scallops so they're a uniform size. Set aside.

2. Add the peanut (or sesame) oil to a heated deep nonstick skillet or wok; sauté the fresh ginger and shallots for 1 to 2 minutes, being careful that the ginger doesn't burn. Add the ground ginger, candied ginger, vinegar, Liquid Aminos, chicken base, and water, and bring to a boil. Remove from heat.

3. Empty the bags of vegetables into a large microwave-safe dish and pour the chicken broth mixture over the vegetables. Cover and microwave on high for 3 to 5 minutes. (The vegetables will continue to steam for a minute or so afterward if the cover remains on the dish.)

4. Bring the skillet or wok back to temperature over medium-high heat. Add the scallops and sauté for 1 minute on each side. Remove the scallops and set aside. Drain the vegetables, reserving the liquid, and transfer to the wok or sauté pan. Stir-fry to bring them up to serving temperature, and add the scallions, if desired.

5. In the meantime, in a small bowl, add the cornstarch to the cold water and whisk to make a slurry. Whisk the slurry into the reserved vegetable liquid; microwave on high for 1 minute. Add the toasted sesame oil, then whisk again. Pour the thickened broth mixture over the vegetables and toss. Add the scallops to the vegetable mixture and stir-fry until the scallops are brought to serving temperature. Serve over rice or pasta.

Tuna Cakes

Serves 9	
Per serving:	
Calories:	92.91
Protein:	7.47 g
Carbohydrates:	9.28 g
Total fat:	3.13 g
Sat. fat:	1.02 g
Cholesterol:	34.14 mg
Sodium:	101.80 mg
Fiber:	0.70 g

2 teaspoons olive oil
2 teaspoons unsalted butter
1 small red onion, chopped
1 small green or red bell pepper, seeded and chopped
Optional: 1 jalapeño chili, seeded and finely chopped
2 cloves garlic, minced
¼ teaspoon dried rosemary
1 teaspoon sweet paprika
1 teaspoon dried basil
1 teaspoon dried parsley
½ teaspoon dried tarragon
½ teaspoon fresh ground white pepper
¼ teaspoon Minor's Crab Base
½ cup water
1 tablespoon lemon juice
½ cup nonfat cottage cheese
1 large egg
1 (6-ounce) can Chicken of the Sea Very Low Sodium Tuna, drained
1 cup bread crumbs
Spectrum Naturals Canola Spray Oil with Butter Flavor

1. Preheat oven to 375°.
2. Bring olive oil and butter to temperature in a nonstick sauté pan over medium heat. Add the onion, bell pepper, and jalapeño, if using; sauté until the onion is transparent. Add the garlic and sauté for 1 minute, being careful not to burn the garlic. Add the rosemary, paprika, basil, parsley, tarragon, and pepper; stir well. Add the Minor's Crab Base; stir well to dissolve into the sautéed vegetable mixture.
3. Add the water and lemon juice to the pan and bring to a boil. Add the cottage cheese and egg to a blender or food processor and pulse to mix. Whisk the cottage cheese mixture into the boiling vegetable mixture in the pan. Reduce heat and simmer until the mixture thickens and the egg is cooked, stirring constantly.
4. Remove from heat and stir in the drained tuna and ¾ cup of the bread crumbs. Treat a square baking pan with the nonstick spray. Pour the mixture into the pan, spreading it out evenly along the bottom. Evenly top with the remaining bread crumbs. Spray the crumbs with the butter-flavored nonstick spray.
5. Bake for 25 to 30 minutes or until the mixture is set and the bread crumbs on top are browned. Cut into 9 pieces.

Baked Seasoned Bread Crumb–Crusted Fish

Spectrum Naturals Canola Spray
  Oil with Butter Flavor
2 large lemons
¼ cup dried bread crumbs
¼ teaspoon onion powder
¼ teaspoon ground fennel seeds
¼ teaspoon freshly ground black
  pepper

⅛ teaspoon celery seeds
⅛ teaspoon dried lemon thyme
⅛ teaspoon dried parsley
⅛ teaspoon salt-free chili powder
1½ pounds halibut fillets

Serves 6	
Per serving:	
Calories:	137.36
Protein:	24.18 g
Carbohydrates:	4.87 g
Total fat:	2.78 g
Sat. fat:	0.39 g
Cholesterol:	36.29 mg
Sodium:	73.38 mg
Fiber:	1.74 g

1. Preheat the oven to 375°. Treat a baking dish with the nonstick spray.
2. Wash the lemons and cut 1 into thin slices; set aside. Grate 1 tablespoon of zest from the second lemon, then juice it into a shallow
   dish; set aside the juice. Combine the grated zest, bread crumbs,
   onion powder, fennel seeds, black pepper, celery seeds, thyme,
   parsley, and chili powder in a small bowl and stir to mix; set aside.
3. Arrange the lemon slices in the bottom of the prepared baking dish.
   Dip the fish pieces in the lemon juice and set them on the lemon
   slices in the baking dish. Sprinkle the bread crumb mixture evenly
   over the fish pieces. Spray the bread crumb topping with a light
   coating of the canola spray oil. Bake until the crumbs are lightly
   browned and the fish is just opaque through, about 10 to 15 minutes.
   (Baking time will depend on the thickness of the fish.) Serve immediately, using the lemon slices as garnish.

Chili-Sauced Stir-Fried Cod and Veggies

Serves 4	
Per serving:	
Calories:	233.66
Protein:	28.54 g
Carbohydrates:	19.97 g
Total fat:	5.18 g
Sat. fat:	0.86 g
Cholesterol:	48.73 mg
Sodium:	385.77 mg
Fiber:	4.97 g

1 tablespoon peanut oil
3 cloves garlic, chopped
1" piece fresh ginger, grated
2 fresh red chilies, sliced
4 heads baby bok choy, halved
2 cups broccoli florets
1 pound cod fillets
1 cup water
2 teaspoons dark brown sugar
½ teaspoon Bragg Liquid Aminos
   or low-sodium soy sauce

½ teaspoon Lea & Perrins
   Worcestershire sauce
2 tablespoons lemon juice
2 tablespoons white wine or sake
1 tablespoon cornstarch mixed
   with 2 tablespoons water
2 green onions, white and green
   parts chopped
Optional: Snipped candied ginger

1. Add the peanut oil to a wok over medium-high heat. Add the garlic, ginger, chilies, bok choy, and broccoli; stir-fry for 1 minute, being careful not to burn the garlic. Remove with a slotted spoon to a serving platter.
2. Wash the cod under cold water and dry between paper towels. Cut into 1" pieces. Add the cod pieces to the now-seasoned peanut oil in the wok; stir-fry for 3 minutes or until opaque, then use tongs or a slotted spoon to transfer them to the platter.
3. Add the water, brown sugar, Liquid Aminos, Worcestershire sauce, lemon juice, and wine (or sake) to the wok; cook, stirring constantly, for 2 minutes to dissolve the sugar. Add the cornstarch slurry and, while continuing to stir, cook for another minute until the sauce thickens. Return the cod, bok choy, and broccoli to the wok, stirring to mix them in with the sauce. Cover and cook for 3 minutes.
4. To serve, divide the mixture over the top of steamed rice. Garnish with the chopped green onion and snipped candied ginger.

Sweet Onion Sole Fillets

2 cups medium-sliced Vidalia
  onions
1 tablespoon balsamic vinegar
2 teaspoons brown sugar
1 pound sole fillets

Spectrum Naturals Extra Virgin
  Olive Spray Oil
1 teaspoon Mrs. Dash Lemon
  Pepper Seasoning Blend or other
  salt-free lemon pepper blend

Serves 4	
Per serving:	
Calories:	208.18
Protein:	23.06 g
Carbohydrates:	13.11 g
Total fat:	6.84 g
Sat. fat:	1.06 g
Cholesterol:	68.00 mg
Sodium:	61.88 mg
Fiber:	1.47 g

1. Preheat oven to 375°.
2. Add the onions to a covered, microwave-safe dish and microwave on high for 5 minutes or until the onions are transparent. Carefully remove the cover (being careful not to burn yourself on the steam) and stir in the vinegar and brown sugar. Cover and microwave on high for an additional 30 seconds. Let stand for several minutes so the onions absorb the flavors. Remove the lid and microwave on high for an additional 30 to 60 seconds to evaporate any excess moisture, watching the onions carefully so they don't burn.
3. Rinse the sole fillets in cold water and pat dry between paper towels. Arrange the fillets on baking sheet treated with the olive spray oil. Lightly spray the top of the fillets with the olive spray oil. Evenly sprinkle the lemon pepper over the fish. Spoon the caramelized onions over the tops of the fillets, pressing them to form a light "crust" over the surface of the fish. Bake for 12 to 15 minutes or until the fish flakes with a fork and the onions darken.

Easy-Baked Cod

Serves 4	
Per serving:	
Calories:	92.93
Protein:	20.18 g
Carbohydrates:	0.00 g
Total fat:	0.76 g
Sat. fat:	0.15 g
Cholesterol:	48.73 mg
Sodium:	61.20 mg
Fiber:	0.00 g

1 pound cod fillets
Spectrum Naturals Extra Virgin
 Olive Spray Oil

1 teaspoon Mrs. Dash Lemon
 Pepper Seasoning Blend or
 other salt-free seasoning blend

1. Preheat oven to 375°.
2. Rinse the cod fillets in cold water and pat dry between paper towels. Arrange the fillets on a baking sheet treated with the olive spray oil. Lightly spray the top of the fillets with the spray oil. Evenly sprinkle the lemon pepper over the fish. Bake for 7 to 10 minutes or until the fish flakes with a fork.

Citrus Pepper Orange Roughy

Serves 4	
Per serving:	
Calories:	117.98
Protein:	16.66 g
Carbohydrates:	0.00 g
Total fat:	5.29 g
Sat. fat:	0.63 g
Cholesterol:	22.67 mg
Sodium:	71.40 mg
Fiber:	0.00 g

4 teaspoons olive oil
4 (4-ounce) orange roughy fillets

2 teaspoons Citrus Pepper
 (page 278)

1. Rinse the fish fillets in cold water and pat dry with paper towels.
2. Bring a large, deep nonstick sauté pan to temperature over medium-high heat. Rub ½ teaspoon of olive oil on each side of each fish fillet. Sprinkle the Citrus Pepper over the curved (or most attractive) side of the fillets. Place the coated fish in the pan, seasoned-side down. Cook for 2 to 3 minutes per side (depending on thickness) until cooked through.

Baked Red Snapper Almandine

1 pound red snapper fillets

4 teaspoons unbleached all-purpose flour

¼ teaspoon freshly ground white or black pepper

¼ teaspoon salt-free chili powder

⅛ teaspoon dried parsley

⅛ teaspoon dried lemon granules, crushed

⅛ teaspoon garlic powder

⅛ teaspoon onion powder

1/16 teaspoon ground coriander

2 teaspoons olive oil

2 tablespoons ground raw almonds

2 teaspoons unsalted butter

1 tablespoon lemon juice

Serves 4	
Per serving:	
Calories:	177.78
Protein:	24.48 g
Carbohydrates:	2.90 g
Total fat:	7.22 g
Sat. fat:	1.94 g
Cholesterol:	47.11 mg
Sodium:	72.91 mg
Fiber:	0.44 g

1. Preheat oven to 375°.
2. Rinse the red snapper fillets and pat dry between layers of paper towels. Add the flour, white (or black) pepper, chili powder, parsley, lemon granules, garlic powder, onion powder, and coriander to a small bowl; mix to combine. Sprinkle the fillets with the seasoned flour, front and back.
3. In an ovenproof nonstick skillet over medium heat, sauté the fillets in the olive oil until they are nicely browned on both sides. Combine the ground almonds and butter in a microwave-safe dish and microwave on high for 30 seconds or until the butter is melted; stir to combine. Pour the almond-butter mixture and lemon juice over the fillets. Bake for 3 to 5 minutes or until the almonds are nicely browned.

❈ Fish Facts

Baking times given for fish dishes assume the fillet is about 1" thick at the thickest part. Fold "tails" or thinner sections under the fish to create an even thickness throughout to help ensure even baking times. That way you'll avoid ending up with some of the fish dry and overdone.

Zesty Fish Fritters

Serves 4	
Per serving:	
Calories:	151.07
Protein:	22.55 g
Carbohydrates:	6.61 g
Total fat:	3.21 g
Sat. fat:	0.63 g
Cholesterol:	101.86 mg
Sodium:	176.25 mg
Fiber:	0.24 g

1 pound cod or other mild white fish fillets

2 tablespoons lemon juice, divided

1 teaspoon garlic powder

½ teaspoon dried ground ginger

½ teaspoon ajowan seeds, pounded or ground with a mortar and pestle

½ teaspoon ground turmeric

½ teaspoon salt-free red chili powder

½ teaspoon ground coriander

¼ teaspoon Garam Masala Spice Blend (page 277)

1 large egg

1 teaspoon canola oil

¼ cup unbleached all-purpose flour

Spectrum Naturals Super Canola Spray Oil

1. Preheat oven to 400°.
2. Rinse the fish in cold water and pat dry. Cut into 1" pieces. Rub the fish with 1 tablespoon of the lemon juice and set aside.
3. In a small bowl, mix the remaining lemon juice with the garlic, ginger, ajowan, turmeric, chili powder, coriander, and garam masala to form a paste. Smear the fish pieces with the spice paste.
4. In a small bowl, beat the egg with the canola oil. Put the flour in another small bowl. Treat a nonstick baking sheet with the nonstick spray. Dip each piece of seasoned fish in the egg mixture, then quickly dip it in the flour so there is just a light dusting of flour on each piece.
5. Arrange the floured fish pieces on the baking tray, leaving some space between them. Spray the tops of the pieces with a light layer of the spray oil. Bake for 10 to 15 minutes, until lightly browned.

❀ Seasonings Primer

Ajowan seed is also called sometimes called ajwain, carom, and lovage. It's a popular spice in Indian cooking, with a flavor similar to thyme. It's often used in bread and bean dishes, too.

Italian-Seasoned Baked Fish

1 pound cod fillets
1 (14.5-ounce) can Muir Glen
  Organic No Salt Added Diced
  Tomatoes
¼ teaspoon dried minced onion
¼ teaspoon onion powder
¼ teaspoon dried minced garlic
¼ teaspoon garlic powder
¼ teaspoon dried basil
¼ teaspoon dried parsley

⅛ teaspoon dried oregano
⅛ teaspoon granulated sugar
⅛ teaspoon dried lemon granules,
  crushed
1/16 teaspoon salt-free chili powder
Optional: Pinch dried red pepper
  flakes
1 tablespoon grated Parmesan
  cheese

Serves 4	
Per serving:	
Calories:	119.86
Protein:	21.53 g
Carbohydrates:	4.32 g
Total fat:	1.14 g
Sat. fat:	0.39 g
Cholesterol:	49.72 mg
Sodium:	121.77 mg
Fiber:	0.83 g

1. Preheat the oven to 375°. Treat a 2- to 3-quart baking pan or casserole dish with nonstick cooking spray.
2. Rinse the cod in cold water and pat dry between paper towels.
3. Add all the ingredients *except* the fish to the prepared baking pan; stir to mix. Arrange the fillets over the tomatoes, folding thin tail ends under to give the fillets even thickness; spoon some of the tomato mixture over the fillets. For fillets about 1" thick, bake uncovered for 20 to 25 minutes or until the fish is opaque and flaky.

❋ Seasoning Sense

Part of the secret of enhancing flavors without salt is to use a variety of complementary seasonings, like the combination of dried ingredients and powders used in the Italian-Seasoned Baked Fish recipe. The sweeter flavors of the powders provide a nice contrast with the chunkier textures created by the dried minced ingredients. Adding some fresh ingredients, too, will enhance this effect even more. In addition, the little bit of dried lemon granules and chili powder further enhance the flavor without directly changing it.

Seafood in Thai-Curry Bean Sauce

Serves 4	
Per serving:	
Calories:	234.58
Protein:	26.81 g
Carbohydrates:	19.48 g
Total fat:	4.18 g
Sat. fat:	0.69 g
Cholesterol:	104.91 mg
Sodium:	193.40 mg
Fiber:	6.53 g

2 teaspoons sesame or canola oil
1 teaspoon curry powder
¼ teaspoon ground black pepper
⅛ teaspoon ground cumin
⅛ teaspoon ground coriander
Pinch dried red pepper flakes
Pinch ground fennel seeds
Pinch ground cloves
Pinch ground mace
1 tablespoon water
1 small sweet onion, finely chopped
2 cloves garlic, minced
1 tablespoon no-salt-added, unsweetened applesauce
¼ cup dry white wine

¼ teaspoon Minor's Low Sodium Chicken Base
¼ cup water
⅛ teaspoon dried lime juice granules, crushed
⅛ teaspoon dried ground lemongrass
¼ packed cup fresh parsley leaves
¼ packed cup fresh basil leaves
1 tablespoon freeze-dried shallots
1⅓ cups canned no-salt-added cannellini (white) beans, drained and rinsed
½ pound shelled and deveined shrimp
½ pound scallops

1. Bring the oil to temperature in a large, deep nonstick sauté pan over medium heat. Add the curry powder, pepper, cumin, coriander, red pepper flakes, fennel seeds, cloves, and mace; sauté for 1 minute. Remove 1 teaspoon of the seasoned oil from the pan and set aside. Add the 1 tablespoon water and bring it to temperature, stirring to mix it with the seasoned oil remaining in the pan. Add the onion and sauté over moderately low heat until the onion is soft. Add the garlic and sauté for 1 minute, being careful not to burn the garlic.

2. Add the applesauce and wine and simmer the mixture until the wine is reduced by half. Add the chicken base and stir to dissolve it and mix it into the onion mixture. Add the ¼ cup water and bring to a boil. Add the lime juice granules, lemongrass, parsley, basil, shallots, and ⅓ cup of the beans. Reduce heat and simmer, stirring, for 1 minute.

3. Transfer the wine-bean mixture to a blender or food processor container; pulse to purée. Pour the wine-bean mixture purée back into the saucepan and add the remaining beans. Simmer to bring the entire mixture to temperature, then keep warm.

4. Wash the shrimp and scallops under cold water. Blot dry between paper towels. Bring a nonstick skillet or sauté pan to temperature over moderately high heat. Add the seasoned oil. When the oil is hot (but not smoking), add the shrimp and sauté for 2 minutes on each side or until cooked through. Using a slotted spoon, transfer the shrimp to a plate and keep warm.

5. Add the scallops to the skillet and sauté for 1 minute on each side or until cooked through. Divide the bean sauce between 4 shallow bowls and arrange the shellfish over the top.

❊ A Fish Story

The cooked weight of seafood can vary considerably, depending on how dry you prefer your fish. Some like fish fillets like tuna or swordfish medium-rare; others prefer well done. The longer the fish cooks, the less it will weigh. Nutritional analysis calculations are based on the amount of seafood called for in the recipe. Therefore, when a recipe calls for precooked seafood, those amounts will be more accurate. Recipes calling for raw seafood weight prior to cooking may actually contain fewer calories than what's indicated in the nutritional analysis, depending on the cooking method used.

Baked Breaded Fish with Lemon

Serves 6	
Per serving:	
Calories:	183.27
Protein:	25.56 g
Carbohydrates:	14.56 g
Total fat:	2.85 g
Sat. fat:	0.40 g
Cholesterol:	36.27 mg
Sodium:	78.88 mg
Fiber:	2.13 g

4 (1-ounce) slices French Bread (page 216)
2 teaspoons Fines Herbes (page 276) or Herbes de Provence (page 276)
¼ teaspoon freshly ground white or black pepper
2 large lemons
1½ pounds halibut fillets
Spectrum Naturals Canola Spray Oil with Butter Flavor

1. Preheat the oven to 375°. Treat a baking dish with nonstick spray.
2. Add the bread, seasoning choice, and pepper to the bowl of a food processor or a blender; process to mix and create bread crumbs. Set aside.
3. Wash the lemons and cut 1 into thin slices. Arrange the slices in the bottom of the prepared dish. Grate the zest from the second lemon, then cut it in half and squeeze the juice into a shallow dish. Combine the grated zest with the prepared bread crumbs; set aside.
4. Rinse the fish fillets in cold water and pat dry with paper towels. Dip the fish pieces in the lemon juice and set them on the lemon slices in the baking dish. Sprinkle the bread crumb mixture evenly over the fish pieces. Lightly mist the bread crumbs with the spray oil. Bake until the crumbs are lightly browned and the fish is opaque, about 10 to 15 minutes. (Baking time will depend on the thickness of the fish.) Serve immediately, using the lemon slices as garnish.

❊ Things Could Get Steamy . . .

Steamers are a convenient way to prepare moist, healthy seafood. Because it circulates the air faster, the Cuisinart Turbo Convection Steamer cooks foods 33 percent faster than conventional models or bamboo steamers. You can use it to prepare an entire meal, and, unlike with conventional steaming methods, you don't have to rearrange or stir the foods during the steaming process. (See Appendix B for company details.)

Easy Oven-Roasted Salmon Steaks

4 (5-ounce) salmon fillets, skin on
2 teaspoons extra-virgin olive oil

1 teaspoon Citrus Pepper
 (page 278)

Serves 4	
Per serving:	
Calories:	240.10
Protein:	25.05 g
Carbohydrates:	0.00 g
Total fat:	14.75 g
Sat. fat:	2.94 g
Cholesterol:	71.40 mg
Sodium:	69.13 mg
Fiber:	0.00 g

1. Preheat the oven to 350°.
2. Rub ½ teaspoon of the olive oil into the flesh side of each salmon fillet. Sprinkle the Citrus Pepper over the olive oil-treated flesh and press it into the fish.
3. Treat an oven-safe baking dish with nonstick spray. Place the fillets skin-side down in the dish. Roast for 25 minutes.

❀ Sodium Slashers

Fresh is usually best, but it isn't always practical. When it comes to seafood, frozen varieties are often frozen in a salty solution (brine). However, even fresh fish may be soaked in brine or sprayed with some other type of preservative to lengthen the shelf life. That's why it's important to wash off the fish using cold, unsoftened water.

CHAPTER 7

Other Meat Entrées

Apple-Spiced Turkey Tenderloins

Serves 4	
Per serving:	
Calories:	197.00
Protein:	26.80 g
Carbohydrates:	16.40 g
Total fat:	2.10 g
Sat. fat:	0.78 g
Cholesterol:	68.00 mg
Sodium:	275.00 mg
Fiber:	6.30 g

2 (8-ounce) turkey tenderloins, cut in half
1 small Granny Smith apple, peeled, cored, and sliced
½ cup apple cider or apple juice
1 tablespoon, plus 2 teaspoons cornstarch
2 teaspoons brown sugar
¼ teaspoon cinnamon
⅛ teaspoon ground ginger
Pinch ground cloves
Pinch ground allspice
Pinch ground nutmeg
½ teaspoon Dijon mustard
¼ teaspoon mustard powder

1. Place the turkey tenderloins between waxed paper or plastic wrap. Use a wooden mallet or rolling pin to pound to ½" thickness. Place in 1 layer in a 10", round Pyrex pie plate. Arrange the apple slices in a circle in the center of the pie plate.
2. In a small bowl, mix together all the remaining ingredients. Pour the mixture over the tenderloins and apple slices. Cover the pie pan tightly with heavy-duty, microwave-safe plastic wrap.
3. Microwave on high for 5 minutes. Turn the plate a half turn. Microwave on high for 4 minutes. Carefully pierce the plastic with a fork to release the steam. Let stand for several minutes and then remove the plastic and serve.

❁ Herb Hints

Rosemary can easily overpower a dish. When left whole in herb-roasted dishes, the flavor isn't as intense (and diners can easily push the rosemary leaves to the side, if they wish). Grinding rosemary in with other spices releases the essential oils and intensifies its flavor. In most cases if you intend to grind it, you'll use about half the amount of dried rosemary called for in a recipe.

Lime-Marinated Grilled Steak

2 tablespoons canola or olive oil
½ cup fresh lime juice
Pinch dried red pepper flakes
½ teaspoon garlic powder
½ teaspoon onion powder
¼ teaspoon ground ginger
⅛ teaspoon dried thyme
⅛ teaspoon salt-free chili powder
Pinch each of ground cinnamon, allspice, and cloves
18-ounce boneless round steak, fat removed
2 teaspoons freshly ground black pepper

Serves 4	
Per serving:	
Calories:	255.00
Protein:	31.00 g
Carbohydrates:	1.00 g
Total fat:	13.20 g
Sat. fat:	3.10 g
Cholesterol:	83.00 mg
Sodium:	60.00 mg
Fiber:	0.00 g

1. In a noncorrosive dish large enough to allow the meat to lie flat, combine the oil, lime juice, red pepper flakes, garlic powder, onion powder, ground ginger, thyme, chili powder, cinnamon, allspice, and cloves. Add steak to the dish, turning it to coat it in the marinade. Cover and refrigerate for 8 hours or overnight. (Turn the meat a few times during this marinating process.)
2. Preheat grill coals to medium-hot (350° to 400°).
3. Remove the meat from the marinade and sprinkle with the black pepper. Grill over direct heat for 4 minutes on one side. Turn and grill for another 2 to 4 minutes, until the meat is cooked to the desired doneness. Transfer to a cutting board or platter and allow the meat to rest for 10 minutes. (Tent with aluminum foil if necessary to maintain meat temperature.) To serve, slice thinly against the grain.

❀ Spice It Up!
If you like spicy hot flavors, substitute a salt-free Thai seasoning or jerk seasoning blend for the spices in the Lime-Marinated Grilled Steak. Both go well with lime juice.

Honey-Grilled Pork Tenderloin

Serves 4	
Per serving:	
Calories:	218.00
Protein:	26.80 g
Carbohydrates:	11.30 g
Total fat:	6.90 g
Sat. fat:	1.80 g
Cholesterol:	83.00 mg
Sodium:	211.00 mg
Fiber:	0.30 g

4 (6-ounce) pork tenderloins, trimmed of all fat
½ cup light beer
3 tablespoons sesame seeds
3 tablespoons honey
¼ teaspoon Dijon mustard
¼ teaspoon mustard powder
½ teaspoon freshly ground black pepper
⅛–¼ teaspoon dried rosemary
2 cloves garlic, minced

1. Add all the ingredients to a heavy-duty, sealable plastic bag, squeezing out as much air as possible when you close the bag. Turn and squeeze the bag to mix the ingredients and cover the meat. Marinate in the refrigerator for at least 2 hours, turning the bag occasionally.
2. Preheat grill coals to medium-hot (350° to 400°).
3. Remove the pork from the marinade and place the tenderloins over indirect heat, grilling the first side for 3 minutes. Use tongs to turn the tenderloins, and continue to grill until the meat temperature registers 155°. (Insert the thermometer probe in the center of a tenderloin at the thickest part.) Transfer to a serving platter and cover with a tent of aluminum foil. Let stand for 10 minutes.
4. While the meat rests, transfer the reserved marinade from the plastic bag to a small saucepan. Bring to a boil over medium-high heat. Reduce heat, but maintain the boil for at least 5 minutes. Be careful that the mixture doesn't burn; add additional water if necessary. Evenly divide the resulting sauce over the grilled meat.

❂ Now You're Smokin'

The Big Easy Gas Grill from Char-Broil has multiple burners, so it's suitable for indirect grilling. That model comes with "SmokerTents" that protect burners and can hold wood chips for smoking foods. Indirect grilling can be done on a charcoal grill if the coals are arranged around the outside edges or to one side of the grill; place the meat so that it's not directly over the heat of the coals.

Roast Beef

2–2¼-pound lean boneless beef
  roast, visible fat removed
1 tablespoon olive or canola oil
1 teaspoon freshly ground black
  pepper
½ teaspoon garlic powder
⅛ teaspoon salt-free chili powder

Pinch dried thyme
1 small white onion, sliced
1 medium-size carrot, peeled and
  sliced
1 large stalk celery, sliced
¼ cup dry red wine
¼ cup water

Serves 8	
Per serving:	
Calories:	252.00
Protein:	22.00 g
Carbohydrates:	18.00 g
Total fat:	10.30 g
Sat. fat:	3.40 g
Cholesterol:	54.00 mg
Sodium:	70.00 mg
Fiber:	0.00 g

1. Preheat oven to 350°. Treat a roasting pan with nonstick spray.
2. Pat the roast dry with paper towels. Add the oil, pepper, garlic powder, chili powder, and thyme to a small bowl and mix well. Rub the oil mixture onto the meat.
3. Place the meat in the center of the prepared pan and arrange the onion, carrot, and celery around it. Pour the wine over the vegetables. Insert the probe of a meat thermometer into the center of thickest part of the roast. Roast, uncovered, to desired doneness. For rare, cook until internal temperature is 125°; for well-done, cook to 170°—approximately 1 to 1¼ hours cooking time.
4. Remove the roast from pan to a cutting board or serving platter. Tent with aluminum foil and allow to rest for 10 to 20 minutes.
5. Remove the vegetables from pan juices with a slotted spoon and discard. Skim off the fat from the pan juices. Serve the juices over the roast.

❀ Think Lean

The onion, carrot, and celery in the Roast Beef recipe are used to flavor the juices. They're discarded because they've absorbed fat that's rendered from the roast. If you want to impart the rich flavor of the pan juices to potatoes or vegetables to be served alongside the roast, roast the potatoes and vegetables on a separate baking sheet. Then, once you've skimmed the fat from the pan juices, toss them with the juices. Return the potatoes and vegetables to the oven while the roast rests.

Braised Herb-Seasoned Pork Chops

Serves 4	
Per serving:	
Calories:	172.00
Protein:	18.00 g
Carbohydrates:	0.00 g
Total fat:	10.00 g
Sat. fat:	4.01 g
Cholesterol:	60.00 mg
Sodium:	46.00 mg
Fiber:	0.00 g

4 (4-ounce) lean, boneless pork loin chops
1 teaspoon olive oil
½ teaspoon marjoram
¼ teaspoon garlic powder
⅛ teaspoon onion powder
⅛ teaspoon freshly ground black pepper
⅛ teaspoon salt-free chili powder
½ cup water

1. Pat the pork chops dry with a paper towel. In a small bowl, mix together the oil, marjoram, garlic powder, onion powder, pepper, and chili powder to form a paste. Rub the mixture onto all sides of the chops.
2. Bring a deep nonstick skillet to temperature over medium-high heat. Add the chops and brown on both sides, cooking for 2 to 3 minutes per side. Add the water and bring to a boil. Reduce heat, cover, and simmer for 1 hour. Serve immediately.

Indoor-Grilled Garlic Sausage

Serves 6	
Per serving:	
Calories:	278.80
Protein:	31.95 g
Carbohydrates:	0.00 g
Total fat:	15.81 g
Sat. fat:	6.01 g
Cholesterol:	98.22 mg
Sodium:	60.07 mg
Fiber:	0.00 g

1 pound lean ground pork
½ pound ground beef sirloin
½ teaspoon garlic powder
1 teaspoon Spice House Salt-Free Bavarian Style Seasoning, Mrs. Dash Garlic and Herb, or The Spice Hunter All Purpose Chef's Blend
Pinch ground cloves
Optional: Pinch dried red pepper flakes
½ teaspoon freshly ground black pepper

1. Preheat indoor grill or bring a large, deep nonstick sauté pan or grill pan to temperature over medium-high heat.
2. Place all the ingredients *except* ¼ teaspoon of the black pepper in a bowl and mix well. Shape into 6 patties. Place the patties on the grill, sprinkling the tops of the patties with the remaining pepper, and close the lid. Grill for 3 to 4 minutes or until the juices run clear.

Slow-Roasted Pork Ribs

1 teaspoon garlic powder

1 teaspoon onion powder

1 teaspoon ground cumin

2 teaspoons salt-free chili powder

2 teaspoons dark brown sugar

1 tablespoon freshly cracked pepper

1/3 teaspoon dried oregano

1/3 teaspoon dried cilantro

2 teaspoons Cascadian Farm frozen Organic Orange Juice Concentrate

1 tablespoon, plus 1 teaspoon water

2 teaspoons lime juice

Dash low-sodium hot red pepper sauce

2 teaspoons olive oil

2-pound rack pork ribs, preferably "3 and down" style

1 tablespoon molasses

2 tablespoons, plus 2 teaspoons low-sodium ketchup

1 tablespoon, plus 1 teaspoon lime juice

1 teaspoon ground cumin

2/3 teaspoon dried cilantro

2 teaspoons salt-free chili powder

1/3 teaspoon salt-free hickory smoke or mesquite base (powder)

Serves 6	
Per serving:	
Calories:	512.56
Protein:	30.72 g
Carbohydrates:	8.70 g
Total fat:	38.79 g
Sat. fat:	14.05 g
Cholesterol:	148.59 mg
Sodium:	131.47 mg
Fiber:	0.12 g

1. Preheat oven to 200°.
2. In the bowl of a food processor fitted with a steel blade or in the jar of a blender, combine the garlic powder, onion powder, cumin, chili powder, brown sugar, pepper, oregano, cilantro, orange juice, water, lime juice, hot red pepper sauce, and olive oil; blend until smooth. Dry the ribs with paper towels, then rub them thoroughly with the paste. Place the ribs on a rack in a large roasting pan and slow-roast for 3 hours or until the meat is tender and pulls easily from the bone. (Ribs can be cooled to room temperature and then refrigerated, covered, for up to 2 days.)
3. In a small bowl, combine the molasses, ketchup, lime juice, cumin, cilantro, chili powder, and hickory smoke (or mesquite base).
4. Place a rack 3" from the broiler. Heat broiler to high. Place the ribs on a baking sheet. Broil for 3 to 5 minutes per side, or until a light crust forms on the surface. Brush the ribs with the molasses mixture and broil for an additional 30 seconds. Use tongs to carefully turn over the ribs and brush that side with the molasses mixture; broil for an additional 30 seconds. To serve, cut the ribs apart between the bones.

Pork Chops and Fruited Veggies Bake

Serves 4	
Per serving:	
Calories:	682.32
Protein:	42.69 g
Carbohydrates:	96.35 g
Total fat:	14.66 g
Sat. fat:	4.98 g
Cholesterol:	108.86 mg
Sodium:	159.64 mg
Fiber:	10.49 g

1 cup baby carrots, washed and peeled
1 (10-ounce) package frozen Cascadian Farm Organic Sliced Peaches, thawed
2 teaspoons brown sugar
¼ teaspoon ground cinnamon
Pinch ground cloves
¼ teaspoon freshly ground black pepper
¼ teaspoon dried thyme
¼ teaspoon dried rosemary

⅛ teaspoon dried oregano
½ teaspoon dried lemon granules
4 (6-ounce) bone-in pork loin chops
8 cloves garlic, crushed
4 large Yukon gold potatoes, washed and sliced
1 (10-ounce) package Cascadian Farms frozen Whole Green Beans, thawed
Spectrum Naturals Extra Virgin Olive Spray Oil

1. Preheat oven to 425°. Treat a large roasting pan or jelly roll pan with nonstick spray.
2. Place the carrots, peaches, brown sugar, cinnamon, and cloves in a medium-sized bowl; stir to mix. Set aside.
3. Mix the pepper, thyme, rosemary, oregano, and lemon granules together and use a mortar and pestle or the back of a spoon to crush them.
4. Rub the pork chops with the garlic. Evenly spread the sliced potatoes and green beans across the prepared baking pan. Place the garlic cloves and pork chops atop the vegetables. Spray lightly with the spray oil. Sprinkle with the herb mixture.
5. Spread the carrot and peach mixture atop the pork chops and vegetables.
6. Bake for 30 minutes or until the meat is tender and the potatoes and carrots are tender.

❀ Fruit Swaps

You can substitute 4 peeled and sliced apples or pears for the peaches in the Pork Chops and Fruited Veggies Bake recipe. If you do, toss the slices with 1 tablespoon of lemon juice before mixing them with the brown sugar, cinnamon, and cloves.

Apricot and Jalapeño-Grilled Lamb Steaks

1 (16-ounce) can apricots in juice
1 tablespoon white wine vinegar
2 teaspoons cornstarch
2 tablespoons seeded and finely
  minced jalapeño peppers
½ cup 100% fruit (no sugar
  added) apricot preserves
2 teaspoons Cascadian Farm
  frozen Organic Orange Juice
  Concentrate

2 tablespoons water
¼ teaspoon mustard powder
8 (5-ounce) lamb sirloin steaks
  (¾" thick)
Spectrum Naturals Extra Virgin Olive
  Spray Oil with Garlic Flavor

Serves 8	
Per serving:	
Calories:	241.00
Protein:	24.50 g
Carbohydrates:	16.60 g
Total fat:	8.00 g
Sat. fat:	2.80 g
Cholesterol:	78.00 mg
Sodium:	100.00 mg
Fiber:	0.30 g

1. Add the juice from the canned apricots, the vinegar, and cornstarch to a small saucepan. Whisk well to remove any lumps. Bring to a boil over medium-high heat. Reduce heat and simmer, stirring constantly for 1 minute or until the mixture thickens. Remove from heat. Finely chop the apricots and add them to the sauce along with the jalapeño. Set aside until ready to serve.
2. Preheat grill coals to medium-hot (350° to 400°).
3. Add the apricot preserves, orange juice concentrate, water, and mustard powder to a microwave-safe bowl; microwave on high for 30 seconds. Whisk the mixture. If it's not yet melted to a spreadable consistency, microwave on high for additional 10-second intervals, stirring after each interval.
4. Pat the steaks dry with paper towels. Lightly spray each side with the garlic-flavored spray. Place the steaks on a grill rack over direct heat. Grill for 3 minutes each side. Baste with the apricot–orange juice mixture and grill for an additional 2 minutes per side, or until cooked to desired doneness. (The direct heat is important at first to sear the meat, but may cause the meat to char once it's basted; if so, use tongs to move the steaks to indirect heat or a spot on the grill that is less hot.) Serve immediately with the apricot-jalapeño sauce.

Veal and Spinach in Lemon Sauce

Serves 6	
Per serving:	
Calories:	194.00
Protein:	20.00 g
Carbohydrates:	5.00 g
Total fat:	11.00 g
Sat. fat:	2.46 g
Cholesterol:	72.00 mg
Sodium:	117.00 mg
Fiber:	2.84 g

3 tablespoons olive or canola oil
1½ pounds lean veal, cut into cubes
1 large white onion, chopped
¼ cup water
1 tablespoon lemon juice
¼ teaspoon freshly ground black pepper
¼ teaspoon fennel seeds, crushed
¼ teaspoon garlic powder

⅛ teaspoon salt-free chili powder
3 green onions, white and green parts chopped
2 (10-ounce) packages frozen spinach
Optional: 1 lemon, cut into 6 wedges

1. Bring oil to temperature over medium-high heat in a large, deep non-stick sauté pan; brown the veal. Add the onion and sauté until transparent. Add the water, lemon juice, pepper, fennel seeds, garlic powder, and chili powder. Bring to a boil, then reduce heat; cover and simmer for 1 hour or until the veal is tender, stirring occasionally and adding more water, if necessary.
2. Add the green onions and spinach. Cover and simmer for 10 minutes. Serve immediately. Garnish with lemon wedges, if desired.

✿ Balsamic Reduction

Add ¼ cup balsamic vinegar to a small sauté pan over medium heat; cook until reduced by half. Remove from heat and dissolve 1 teaspoon of brown sugar into the vinegar reduction. Add freshly ground black pepper and stir well. As is, this reduction is surprisingly good over fresh strawberries or vanilla ice cream—or both! To serve as a steak or other meat sauce, omit the brown sugar and stir in 2 teaspoons of American Spoon Foods jalapeño jelly or berry jam or a teaspoon of butter instead. A little goes a long way, so this will make 4 to 8 servings, depending on your tastes and usage.

Sweet and Spicy Kielbasa

1 teaspoon bourbon
Pinch dried red pepper flakes
1 pound pork shoulder
½ pound beef chuck
1 teaspoon freshly ground black
   pepper

½ teaspoon ground allspice
1 teaspoon garlic powder
⅛ teaspoon ground mustard
1 teaspoon brown sugar

Serves 6	
Per serving:	
Calories:	283.61
Protein:	31.95 g
Carbohydrates:	0.75 g
Total fat:	15.81 g
Sat. fat:	6.01 g
Cholesterol:	98.22 mg
Sodium:	60.37 mg
Fiber:	0.00 g

1. Preheat indoor grill or bring a large, deep nonstick sauté pan or grill pan to temperature over medium-high heat.
2. Put the bourbon in a microwave-safe bowl and add the pepper flakes; microwave on high for 15 seconds or until the mixture is hot. In a large bowl, combine the seasoned bourbon with all the remaining ingredients *except* ¼ teaspoon of the black pepper; mix well. Shape into 6 patties. Place the patties on the grill, sprinkling the tops of the patties with the remaining pepper, and close the lid. Grill for 3 to 4 minutes or until the juices run clear.

❀ Beef Broth

Some chefs contend that the addition of oven-roasted beef bones is essential for a hearty beef broth. Adding the Minor's Low Sodium Beef Base saves you that time and hassle when you make the Easy Slow-Cooked "Roast" Beef recipe; the broth that results is full-bodied and delicious. Strain any fat from that broth, or even better, refrigerate the broth overnight and then remove and discard the hardened fat. The broth can be kept for 1 or 2 days in the refrigerator, or frozen up to 3 months. On average, the nutritional analysis for each ½-cup serving of the resulting beef broth will be: Calories: 2.14; Protein: 1.80 g; Carbohydrates: 0.21 g; Total Fat: 0.42 g; Sat. Fat: 0.15 g; Cholesterol: 4.39 mg; Sodium: 21.28 mg; Fiber: 0.00 g.

Beef Fillet

Serves 8	
Per serving:	
Calories:	157.07
Protein:	24.01 g
Carbohydrates:	0.84 g
Total fat:	6.06 g
Sat. fat:	2.56 g
Cholesterol:	66.94 mg
Sodium:	45.43 mg
Fiber:	0.00 g

2-pound fillet of beef, trimmed and tied
1½ teaspoons unsalted butter, at room temperature
1½ teaspoons olive oil
1½ teaspoons coarsely ground black pepper

2 teaspoons sweet paprika
2 tablespoons garlic powder
1½ teaspoons onion powder
½ teaspoon cayenne pepper
⅓ teaspoon dried oregano
⅓ teaspoon dried thyme

1. Preheat the oven to 500°. Treat a baking sheet or a roasting rack set in a roasting pan with nonstick spray.
2. Pat the outside of the meat dry with a paper towel. Place the meat on a piece of heavy-duty aluminum foil large enough to hold the fillet. Set aside to come to room temperature while you perform the other steps.
3. In a small bowl, mix together the unsalted butter and olive oil.
4. In another small bowl, combine all the remaining dry ingredients; mix well.
5. Use your hands to spread the butter–olive oil mixture over the entire surface of the meat. Sprinkle the dry seasoning mixture evenly over the entire surface of the meat, patting it into the meat. Move the fillet to the prepared baking sheet or roasting rack. Insert the probe of a meat thermometer into the center of thickest part of the fillet. Roast, uncovered, to desired doneness. (Keep in mind that the temperature of the fillet will rise by a few degrees while it rests in step 6.)
6. Remove the beef from the oven, and place it under an aluminum foil "tent" that is crimped tightly to the pan. Allow the meat to rest at room temperature for 20 minutes. Remove the tent and the strings holding the meat together; use a serrated knife to slice the fillet into 16 equal-sized pieces.

❀ Keep It Clean

Be sure your oven is very clean when you set it to use high temperatures; otherwise, the high temperatures will cause it to smoke.

Grilled Lamb Steaks

4 (5-ounce) lean lamb sirloin
  steaks (¾" thick)

2 teaspoons olive oil
1 clove garlic, crushed

1. Preheat grill coals to medium-hot (350° to 400°).
2. Pat the lamb steaks dry with a paper towel. Add the olive oil and garlic to a microwave-safe bowl; microwave on high for 20 seconds. Rub the garlic-infused olive oil into all sides of the steaks. Rub the softened garlic clove across the top of each steak.
3. Place the steaks on grill rack over direct heat. Grill for 5 minutes on each side or desired doneness. (The direct heat is important at first to sear the meat, but if it starts to char, use tongs to move the steaks to indirect heat or to a spot on the grill that is less hot.)

Serves 4	
Per serving:	
Calories:	357.61
Protein:	29.58 g
Carbohydrates:	0.25 g
Total fat:	25.61 g
Sat. fat:	10.11 g
Cholesterol:	112.20 mg
Sodium:	88.53 mg
Fiber:	0.02 g

Minted Bread Sauce

¾ cup fresh mint
¼ cup stale bread crumbs
4 teaspoons extra-virgin olive oil

⅛ teaspoon freshly ground pepper
1 teaspoon red wine vinegar
¼ teaspoon Dijon mustard

Add the mint and bread crumbs to the bowl of a food processor. Pulse to finely chop the mint. Add the olive oil, pepper, vinegar, and mustard. Pulse to mix thoroughly. The flavor improves with time as the sauce sits, so prepare it at least 30 minutes in advance and allow it to rest in the covered food processor. If the sauce mixture is too tight, add water 1 teaspoon at a time to loosen it.

Serves 4	
Per serving:	
Calories:	61.64
Protein:	1.03 g
Carbohydrates:	3.43 g
Total fat:	5.14 g
Sat. fat:	0.66 g
Cholesterol:	0.03 mg
Sodium:	192.04 mg
Fiber:	0.95 g

South of the Border Sausage

Serves 16	
Per serving:	
Calories:	135.43
Protein:	15.43 g
Carbohydrates:	0.00 g
Total fat:	7.72 g
Sat. fat:	2.90 g
Cholesterol:	45.33 mg
Sodium:	27.20 mg
Fiber:	0.00 g

2 pounds ground pork shoulder
1 teaspoon ground black pepper
1 teaspoon dried parsley
1 teaspoon salt-free chili powder
1 teaspoon garlic powder
1 teaspoon onion powder
½ teaspoon paprika
⅛ teaspoon dried red pepper flakes, crushed
⅛ teaspoon Mexican oregano, crushed
Pinch ground cinnamon
Pinch ground cloves

Add all ingredients to a bowl and mix until well blended. The traditional preparation method calls for putting the sausage mixture in casings; however, it works equally well when it's shaped into 16 small sausage patties and broiled or grilled, or sautéed to be combined with the ingredients in other dishes.

Sweet Pepper and Fennel Sausage

Serves 8	
Per serving:	
Calories:	277.10
Protein:	30.95 g
Carbohydrates:	1.60 g
Total fat:	15.45 g
Sat. fat:	5.79 g
Cholesterol:	90.67 mg
Sodium:	54.66 mg
Fiber:	0.07 g

1 teaspoon fennel seeds, crushed
⅛ teaspoon salt-free chili powder
2 pounds ground pork butt
½ teaspoon freshly ground black pepper
⅛ teaspoon mustard powder
Pinch cayenne pepper
2 teaspoons crushed garlic
¼ cup finely minced roasted red pepper, skin removed (see instructions for roasting peppers on page 58)
½ teaspoon honey

Toast the fennel seeds and cayenne pepper in a nonstick skillet over medium heat until the seeds just begin to darken, about 2 minutes, stirring constantly. Cool, then grind using a spice grinder or mortar and pestle. Add to a bowl along with the remaining ingredients and mix until well blended. Shape into 8 patties. Prepare by grilling, broiling, or sautéing, cooking until the juices run clear.

Lamb Stew

2½ pounds lean boneless lamb
  chops, cut into 1" chunks
1 tablespoon canola oil
3 large white or yellow onions,
  quartered
¼ teaspoon garlic powder
Pinch dried red pepper flakes
4 large carrots, peeled and sliced
  into chunks
4 cups water

4 large potatoes, peeled and cut
  into large dice
1 tablespoon unsalted butter
1 teaspoon red wine or balsamic
  vinegar
1 teaspoon dried parsley
½ teaspoon dried thyme
¼ teaspoon mustard powder
¼ teaspoon freshly ground pepper

Serves 4	
Per serving:	
Calories:	693.00
Protein:	48.80 g
Carbohydrates:	50.73 g
Total fat:	34.50 g
Sat. fat:	16.46 g
Cholesterol:	217.56 mg
Sodium:	160.71 mg
Fiber:	6.80 g

1. Bring a large, deep nonstick sauté pan to temperature over medium-high heat. Add the oil and once it's almost smoking, add the lamb and brown on all sides. Remove the lamb with a slotted spoon and keep warm. Add the onion and sauté until transparent. Stir in the garlic powder and dried pepper flakes. Add the carrots, and return lamb to the pan along with the water; bring to a boil. Lower heat, cover, and simmer for 1 hour.
2. Add the potatoes and simmer for a minimum of 1 more hour, or until the meat and potatoes are tender.
3. Allow the stew to rest for 5 to 10 minutes. Skim off any fat from the top of the stew. Either pour off some of the broth or ladle it into a small saucepan over medium-high heat. Bring the broth to a boil, then whisk in the butter, vinegar, parsley, thyme, mustard powder, and pepper. Pour the seasoned broth over the stew and stir to mix. Serve immediately.

❀ Onion Yields
On average, 1 tablespoon of onion powder is the equivalent of 1 medium-size onion, or 1 cup of chopped onion or ½ cup of minced onion. If using dried minced onion, plan on using one-fourth of what's called for in the recipe if replacing chopped onion and half if replacing minced.

Turkey Patties with Cranberry Sauce

Serves 4	
Per serving:	
Calories:	163.75
Protein:	27.46 g
Carbohydrates:	6.59 g
Total fat:	2.37 g
Sat. fat:	0.63 g
Cholesterol:	65.77 mg
Sodium:	244.45 mg
Fiber:	0.59 g

1 tablespoon Cascadian Farm Organic Cranberry Frozen Concentrated Juice Cocktail
1 tablespoon water
1 teaspoon dried orange granules, crushed
1 tablespoon red currant jelly
¼ teaspoon Dijon mustard

1 pound lean ground turkey
1 tablespoon freeze-dried green onion or shallot
1 teaspoon garlic powder
¼ teaspoon freshly ground black pepper
Pinch ground cloves

1. Prepare the cranberry sauce by adding the cranberry juice cocktail concentrate, water, orange granules, and red currant jelly to a small microwave-safe bowl; microwave on high for 30 seconds. Stir to mix. Whisk in the Dijon mustard.
2. Mix the ground turkey with the onion (or shallot), garlic powder, pepper, and cloves. Shape into 4 patties. Either bring a nonstick grill pan to temperature over medium-high heat or preheat a George Foreman–style indoor grill. Fry or grill the patties until the juices run clear. Serve hot with the cranberry sauce drizzled over the top of the patties.

❋ Sauce Savvy

Commercial sauces are often sodium-laden preparations used to disguise rather than enhance the flavors of processed foods. Sugar is also often added to mask flavors. When buying no-salt-added or low-sodium commercial sauces, choose those with less than 5 grams of sugar per serving.

Jumbo Hamburger-Tofu Cheeseburgers

8 ounces firm tofu
¼ cup low-salt ketchup
½ teaspoon onion powder
1 teaspoon garlic powder
¼ teaspoon cracked pepper
¼ pound ground round

¼ pound ground turkey
4 (½-ounce) slices Cabot 50%
    Light Jalapeno Cheddar Cheese
4 reduced-sodium, reduced-calorie
    hamburger buns
8 large iceberg lettuce leaves

Serves 4	
Per serving:	
Calories:	337.52
Protein:	27.00 g
Carbohydrates:	25.75 g
Total fat:	16.35 g
Sat. fat:	5.36 g
Cholesterol:	51.08 mg
Sodium:	334.84 mg
Fiber:	4.59 g

1. In a small bowl, mix together the crumbled tofu, ketchup, onion powder, garlic powder, and pepper. Allow 15 minutes or longer for the ketchup and seasonings to be absorbed by the tofu. Add the ground meats to the bowl and mix well.
2. Preheat an indoor grill. Shape the tofu-meat mixture into 4 patties and grill until the juices run clear. The grilling time will depend on whether or not you're using a grill with a "lid" or grilling one side at a time.
3. Lift the lid of the grill and blot the tops of the burgers with paper towels to absorb any fat that hasn't run off during the grilling process. Place the cheese slices on top of the burgers and allow time for the cheese to melt.
4. Place a lettuce leaf on top of each bottom half of the buns. Use a heat-safe spatula or tongs to transfer the burgers to the buns. Top each burger with the remaining lettuce and top half of the buns.

❀ Mushroom Burger Alternative

A fast-food, quarter-pound cheeseburger usually has more than 500 calories and a whopping 1,000 or more milligrams of sodium. Combining tofu with the meat is a way to prepare a huge hamburger and cut the fat and sodium. Cooking your burgers using this method improves the flavor, so even the fussiest eater in your family won't notice the difference. If tofu isn't your thing, use 1 cup of finely chopped, steamed, and well-drained mushroom pieces instead. Doing so will reduce the calories to 265.83, the fat to 11.59 grams, and the sodium to 327.68 milligrams.

Quick Seasoned Jumbo Hamburgers

Serves 4	
Per serving:	
Calories:	186.13
Protein:	29.58 g
Carbohydrates:	0.28 g
Total fat:	6.56 g
Sat. fat:	2.48 g
Cholesterol:	84.17 mg
Sodium:	70.40 mg
Fiber:	0.00 g

½ pound lean ground sirloin
¼ pound boneless, skinless chicken breast, ground
¼ pound boneless, skinless turkey breast, ground

1 teaspoon Mrs. Dash Steak Grilling Blend or Mesquite Grilling Blend
¼ teaspoon brown sugar

1. In a mixing bowl, combine all the ingredients until well mixed. Form into 4 equal-sized patties.
2. Pan-fry in a nonstick grill pan or prepare in a covered indoor grill (such as a George Foreman–style indoor grill). The sausage is done when the juices run clear.

Easy Italian-Seasoned Turkey Sausage

Serves 8	
Per serving:	
Calories:	84.93
Protein:	9.95 g
Carbohydrates:	0.00 g
Total fat:	4.71 g
Sat. fat:	1.28 g
Cholesterol:	45.03 mg
Sodium:	53.58 mg
Fiber:	0.00 g

1 pound lean ground turkey

1½ teaspoons Spice Hunter Italian Pizza Seasoning or Mrs. Dash Classic Italiano Seasoning Blend

1. In a mixing bowl, combine the ground turkey with your choice of seasoning blend until well mixed. Form into 8 equal-sized patties.
2. Pan-fry in a nonstick grill pan or prepare in a covered indoor grill (such as a George Foreman–style indoor grill). The sausage is done when the juices run clear.

Liverwurst

Unbleached muslin
1 pound fresh pork liver
1 pound lean beef round steak,
    trimmed of any fat
1 large white onion, finely diced
3 tablespoons nonfat dry milk
1 teaspoon freshly fine-ground
    white pepper
2 teaspoons paprika

1 teaspoon granulated sugar
½ teaspoon marjoram
½ teaspoon finely ground coriander
¼ teaspoon mace
¼ teaspoon allspice
¼ teaspoon ground cardamom
¼ teaspoon mustard powder
⅛ teaspoon dried lemon granules,
    crushed

Serves 6	
Per serving:	
Calories:	218.16
Protein:	33.78 g
Carbohydrates:	4.51 g
Total fat:	6.22 g
Sat. fat:	2.07 g
Cholesterol:	272.64 mg
Sodium:	123.35 mg
Fiber:	0.00 g

1. In place of casings, prepare a piece of unbleached muslin about 12" long and 8" wide. Fold the muslin lengthwise and tightly stitch a seam across 1 of the short ends and continue along the open side. Leave a seam of about ⅛" from the edge of the material. Turn the muslin casing so that the stitching is on the inside. Set it aside until you are ready to stuff it.

2. Run the liver and round steak through a meat grinder with the fine disk. Mix well to combine the liver and beef. Transfer the ground meat to a bowl, sprinkle the remaining ingredients over the ground meat, and mix thoroughly.

3. Pack the mixture into the muslin casing. (It's easier to get the meat packed to the bottom of the casing if you first fold the open end down over itself.) Firmly pack the meat into the casing. Either stitch the open end closed or secure it with a twist tie, butcher's twine, or cotton cord.

4. In a large kettle, bring enough water to a boil to cover the liverwurst in the muslin packet by 2 or 3". Place a weight—such as a heavy plate—on it to keep it submerged. Bring the water to a boil; reduce the heat, cover, and simmer for 3 hours.

5. Either transfer the muslin packet to a pan of ice water or drain the hot water from the pan and replace it with an equal quantity of ice water. Let the liverwurst cool, then refrigerate it overnight. Remove the muslin casing and slice the liverwurst into 4-ounce portions to serve.

Sausage Gravy

Serves 4	
Per serving:	
Calories:	102.43
Protein:	12.53 g
Carbohydrates:	7.35 g
Total fat:	2.24 g
Sat. fat:	0.62 g
Cholesterol:	15.78 mg
Sodium:	73.33 mg
Fiber:	0.05 g

1 cup nonfat cottage cheese
1 cup skim milk
¼ cup instant nonfat dry milk
⅛ pound Peppery Turkey Sausage (page 68)
⅛ teaspoon mustard powder

Pinch dried lemon granules, crushed
2 teaspoons olive oil
1 tablespoon unbleached all-purpose flour

1. In a blender or food processor container, combine the cottage cheese, skim milk, and dry milk; process until smooth. Set aside.
2. In a large, deep nonstick sauté pan, fry the sausage until done, breaking it into small pieces with a heat-safe spatula as you fry it. Add the mustard powder, lemon granules, and olive oil; mix well and heat until sizzling. Add the flour, stirring constantly to create a roux (the thickening agent). Gradually stir in some of the cottage cheese mixture, using the back of spatula or a whisk to blend it with the roux; stir constantly to avoid lumps. Once you have about ½ cup of the cottage cheese mixture blended into the roux, you can add the remaining amount.
3. Continue to cook, stirring constantly, until the mixture begins to steam. Lower the heat and allow the mixture to simmer (being careful that it doesn't come to a boil) until the gravy reaches the desired consistency.

❋ Savory Sweet Sausage

A touch of sugar or other sweet ingredients added to sausage before it's cooked not only sweetens the meat, it also aids in the caramelization process that takes place when meat is seared at high temperatures. The "sugar" in such recipes can be a substitute of honey or fruit, or a sweet low-sodium condiment like American Spoon Foods (see Appendix B) Red Spoon Peppers, Mango Habanero Salsa, or Kiwi Lime Salsa Verde.

Seasoned Pork Roast

½ pound pork loin roast
½ cup dry white wine
1 tablespoon lemon juice
1 teaspoon olive oil
⅛ cup Mr. Spice honey mustard
sauce

1 tablespoon minced shallots
½ teaspoon onion powder
¼ teaspoon garlic powder
¼ teaspoon dried thyme
⅛ teaspoon ground black pepper

Serves 4	
Per serving:	
Calories:	113.21
Protein:	12.21 g
Carbohydrates:	2.39 g
Total fat:	3.59 g
Sat. fat:	1.16 g
Cholesterol:	33.45 mg
Sodium:	31.07 mg
Fiber:	0.06 g

1. Pat the pork loin with paper towels to remove any excess moisture. In a heavy, freezer-style, sealable plastic bag, combine all the remaining ingredients; turn the bag until the ingredients are well mixed. Add the meat to the marinade and turn the bag to coat the meat evenly. Place the bag in the refrigerator. (Note: The longer you marinate the meat, the more intense the sauerbraten-style flavor of the meat. Pork loin is already tender, so you're marinating the meat only to impart the flavors.)
2. Preheat oven to 350°. Treat the rack of a roasting pan with nonstick spray.
3. Remove the meat from marinade and place it on the prepared rack in the roasting pan. Roast until a meat thermometer reads 150° to 170°, depending on your preference. Tent the roast with aluminum foil and let "rest" for 10 minutes before carving.

❀ Paprika Primer

Paprika sold in the supermarket is mild in flavor, usually good mostly for adding color to a dish. You can alter the flavor of a dish by getting one of the paprika varieties from a specialty shop, like the Spice House (see Appendix B). Varieties include Budapest Exquisite Sweet, California (mild with a deep red color), Hungarian Sweet, Hungarian Half Sharp (slightly spicier), Smoked Spanish Sweet, and Smoked Spanish Hot Paprikas.

CHAPTER 8
Casseroles and One-Dish Meals

Italian Casserole

Serves 4	
Per serving:	
Calories:	353.19
Protein:	16.73 g
Carbohydrates:	25.11 g
Total fat:	20.29 g
Sat. fat:	8.85 g
Cholesterol:	118.39 mg
Sodium:	441.98 mg
Fiber:	2.67 g

¼ pound ground pork
1 teaspoon onion powder
½ teaspoon Mrs. Dash Classic Italiano Seasoning Blend
½ teaspoon Mrs. Dash Garlic and Herb Seasoning Blend
1 (14.5-ounce) can Muir Glen Organic No Salt Added Diced Tomatoes

¼ cup whole-milk ricotta cheese
¼ cup cottage cheese
2 ounces provolone cheese, shredded or cut into small pieces
1 large egg, beaten
2 cups spinach noodles, cooked

1. Preheat oven to 350°. Treat a casserole dish with nonstick spray.
2. Bring a small nonstick sauté pan treated with nonstick spray to temperature over medium-high heat. Add the ground pork. Sprinkle with the onion powder and seasoning blends. Pan-fry until cooked through. (At this point you can blot the pork with paper towels to remove excess fat; however, the nutritional analysis allows for the fat.)
3. Add the cooked pork, tomatoes, cheeses, and egg to a large bowl; stir to combine. Fold the cooked noodles into the mixture, making sure the noodles are completely coated. Pour the mixture into the prepared casserole dish. Bake for 45 minutes or until the mixture is heated through and set and the cheese is melted.

❋ Cheese, Please

Cheese can be a valuable source of calcium—if chosen wisely. Avoid processed cheese; it has a much higher sodium content. Natural cheese is best. Think of its use in a dish as that of a condiment to enhance the flavor rather than as the main ingredient.

Palate Pleasin' Pork Potpie

¼ cup Cascadian Farm Organic Frozen Apple Juice Concentrate

1 teaspoon Minor's Pork Base

½ teaspoon Minor's Roasted Mirepoix Flavor Concentrate

Boiling water

¼ cup chopped prunes, pitted

¼ cup chopped dried apricots

¼ cup seedless raisins

12 juniper berries, lightly crushed

½ teaspoon dried thyme

½ teaspoon dried parsley

⅛ teaspoon freshly ground black pepper

2 pounds lean boneless pork, cut into small cubes

1 large sweet onion, chopped

2 cloves garlic, minced

1 stalk celery, minced

4 carrots, peeled and chopped

4 large potatoes, peeled and diced

1 (10-ounce) package Cascadian Farm Frozen Petite Sweet Peas, thawed

1 cup unbleached all-purpose flour

Pinch dried lemon granules, crushed

½ teaspoon garlic powder

¼ teaspoon onion powder

1 large egg, beaten

1 teaspoon low-salt baking powder

2 tablespoons canola or light olive oil

⅓ cup skim milk

Optional: Fresh chopped parsley

Serves 8	
Per serving:	
Calories:	609.07
Protein:	40.29 g
Carbohydrates:	64.92 g
Total fat:	20.58 g
Sat. fat:	4.78 g
Cholesterol:	116.47 mg
Sodium:	421.28 mg
Fiber:	6.78 g

1. Preheat oven to 300°.
2. Add the apple juice concentrate, pork base, and roasted mirepoix flavor concentrate to a heat-safe measuring cup. Add 1 cup boiling water and stir to mix. Place the prunes, apricots, raisins, juniper berries, thyme, parsley, and pepper in a bowl. Pour the apple juice mixture over the fruit and seasonings in the bowl; cover and set aside for 20 minutes.
3. In a large Dutch oven treated with nonstick spray, add the pork, onion, garlic, celery, carrots, and potatoes. Pour the fruit and seasoning mixture into the pan over the pork and vegetables. Add enough boiling water to bring the water level up to the halfway mark of the pan. Cover and bake for 1½ hours.
4. Remove the pan from the oven. Remove the cover. (The meat should be tender at this point. If not, return the pan to the oven for another

(continues on page 142)

Palate Pleasin' Pork Potpie (continued)

30 minutes before you proceed.) Add the peas, gently stirring to combine with the other ingredients. Increase oven temperature to 350°.

5. Add the flour, lemon granules, garlic and onion powders, egg, baking powder, oil, and skim milk to a bowl. Use a fork to combine and form a dough; do not overmix the ingredients. Use a tablespoon to drop 8 mounds of dough over the top of the pork mixture. (Allow some space between each dough mound so that the edges aren't touching.) Cover and return to the oven for 30 to 35 minutes, or until the dough is cooked.

6. Remove the pan from the oven and uncover; let rest for 5 to 10 minutes. Ladle into serving bowls. Serve immediately, topped with freshly ground pepper. Garnish with fresh parsley, if desired.

❀ Food Facts
It's a fallacy that you sear meat before roasting it to "seal in the juices." You sear the meat to add the additional layer of flavor that results from caramelizing the meat over a high temperature. Because Minor's Pork Base and other meat bases are made from highly concentrated roasted meat and meat juices, you get the benefit of pan-seared flavor without the fuss.

Quick Summer Luncheon Plate

1 (6-ounce) can Chicken of the Sea Very Low Sodium Tuna, drained

1 (15-ounce) can Eden Organics No Salt Added Cannellini (white kidney) Beans, drained and rinsed

1 teaspoon capers, nonpareil in brine, drained, rinsed, and crushed or minced

1 small red onion, ½ minced and ½ thinly sliced

2 large tomatoes, peeled, seeded, and chopped

1 tablespoon balsamic or red wine vinegar

2 tablespoons extra-virgin olive oil

1 tablespoon water

⅛ teaspoon mustard powder

⅛ teaspoon fresh ground black pepper

Pinch dried red pepper flakes, crushed

3 fresh basil leaves, minced

1 tablespoon minced fresh parsley

2 cups salad greens, torn into bite-size pieces

2 teaspoons grated Parmesan cheese

Serves 2	
Per serving:	
Calories:	442.83
Protein:	34.12 g
Carbohydrates:	41.15 g
Total fat:	17.18 g
Sat. fat:	2.25 g
Cholesterol:	38.82 mg
Sodium:	214.99 mg
Fiber:	11.72 g

1. Add the drained tuna to a medium-size bowl and break it into bite-size pieces with a fork. Add the beans, capers, minced onion, and tomatoes; mix well.

2. In a small jar, combine the red wine vinegar, oil, water, mustard power, pepper, dried pepper flakes, basil, and parsley; cover the jar and shake until the dressing is emulsified. Pour the dressing over the tuna mixture; mix well and set aside.

3. Place 1 cup of the salad greens on each of 2 serving plates. Top with the onion slices and tuna mixture. Grind some additional black pepper over the tops of the salads, if desired, and top each with 1 teaspoon of freshly grated Parmesan cheese; serve immediately.

❋ Shop Wisely

Avoid the expensive varieties of tuna packed in olive oil. Instead, opt for no-salt-added varieties. Tuna is a salt-water fish, so it has a naturally salty flavor. Buying tuna packed in water lets you choose the amount and quality of olive oil you add.

Boiled Seafood Plates

Serves 4	
Per serving:	
Calories:	467.12
Protein:	36.94 g
Carbohydrates:	67.03 g
Total fat:	2.12 g
Sat. fat:	0.30 g
Cholesterol:	116.17 mg
Sodium:	280.17 mg
Fiber:	9.36 g

6 cups water
2 tablespoons dried minced garlic
2 tablespoons salt-free Old Bay
   Seasoning (page 274)
2 (12-ounce) bottles or cans of
   beer
½ cup fresh lemon juice
1–4 tablespoons (to taste) granulated sugar
4 medium-size red potatoes
1 jumbo Vidalia onion, sliced

1 (10-ounce) package Cascadian
   Farm Frozen Gardener's Blend
   Vegetables
1 (10-ounce) package Cascadian
   Farm frozen California Blend
   Vegetables
2 (4-ounce) frozen orange roughy
   fillets
½ pound scallops
½ pound frozen shrimp
1 large lemon, cut into 4 wedges

1. Bring the water to a boil in a Dutch oven or stockpot. Add the garlic, Old Bay, beer, and lemon juice. Add the sugar 1 tablespoon at a time, tasting after each to determine preferred sweetness level. (The liquid will still taste somewhat bitter and spicy.) Bring the stock to a boil, turn off the burner, and let sit for 30 minutes.

2. Bring the cooking liquid to a boil a second time. Add the potatoes and onion, reduce heat, and let simmer until they are almost done.

3. Add the frozen vegetables. Allow the cooking liquid to return to a simmer, then adjust heat to lowest setting and let simmer for 10 minutes, stirring occasionally.

4. Rinse the seafood under cold, running water to remove any frost crystals, if necessary. Add the frozen fish fillets and let simmer for about 5 minutes. Add the scallops and simmer for an additional 5 minutes.

5. Add the frozen shrimp; simmer until the shrimp is thawed, about 2 minutes.

6. Use a slotted spoon to transfer a potato to each serving plate; slice the potatoes in half or into wedges. Use the slotted spoon to divide the seafood and remaining vegetables between the 4 plates. Squeeze a lemon wedge over each, and serve.

Slow-Cooked Venison

2¼-pound lean venison roast, trimmed of fat and cut into pieces
Water, as needed
¼ teaspoon Minor's Low Sodium Beef Base

⅛ teaspoon Minor's Roasted Mirepoix Flavor Concentrate
1 tablespoon cider vinegar

Serves 8	
Per serving:	
Calories:	179.99
Protein:	34.28 g
Carbohydrates:	0.09 g
Total fat:	3.63 g
Sat. fat:	1.41 g
Cholesterol:	126.85 mg
Sodium:	69.74 mg
Fiber:	0.00 g

1. Put the venison in a ceramic-lined slow cooker, add enough water to cover the roast, and set the cooker on high. Dissolve the bases in the vinegar and add to the cooker. Once the mixture begins to boil, reduce temperature to low. Allow the meat to simmer for 8 hours or until tender.
2. Drain off and discard the resulting broth from the meat. Remove any remaining fat from the meat and discard that as well. Weigh the meat and separate it into 4-ounce servings. The meat can be kept for 1 or 2 days in the refrigerator, or freeze portions for use later.

Easy Slow-Cooked "Roast" Beef

2¼-pound London broil roast, trimmed of fat and cut into pieces
Water, as needed
½ teaspoon Minor's Low Sodium Beef Base

⅛ teaspoon Minor's Roasted Mirepoix Flavor Concentrate
½ tablespoon dried minced onion
½ teaspoon dried minced garlic

Serves 8	
Per serving:	
Calories:	246.26
Protein:	40.45 g
Carbohydrates:	0.16 g
Total fat:	8.10 g
Sat. fat:	2.88 g
Cholesterol:	102.10 mg
Sodium:	65.37 mg
Fiber:	0.00 g

1. Put the roast and all other ingredients into a ceramic-lined slow cooker, add enough water to cover the roast, and set the cooker on high. Once the mixture begins to boil, stir to dissolve the bases; reduce temperature to low. Allow the meat to simmer for 8 hours or until tender.
2. Remove the meat from the slow cooker and discard the resulting broth (or save it for later use). Remove any remaining fat from the meat and discard that as well. Weigh the meat and separate it into 4-ounce servings. The meat can be kept for 1 or 2 days in the refrigerator, or freeze portions for use later.

Venison and Veggie Stovetop Casserole

Serves 4	
Per serving:	
Calories:	411.31
Protein:	38.18 g
Carbohydrates:	45.54 g
Total fat:	5.05 g
Sat. fat:	2.09 g
Cholesterol:	129.69 mg
Sodium:	126.26 mg
Fiber:	6.02 g

1 teaspoon olive oil
1 teaspoon butter
1 small sweet onion, chopped
½ cup Muir Glen Organic No Salt
   Added Tomato Purée
2 cloves garlic, minced
¼ teaspoon Minor's Low Sodium
   Beef Base
¾ cup dry red wine
2 tablespoons red currant jelly
½ cup water
⅛ cup lemon juice
1 tablespoon cornstarch
Optional: ¼ teaspoon granulated
   sugar
¼ teaspoon dried parsley

⅛ teaspoon salt-free chili powder
⅛ teaspoon mustard powder
⅛ teaspoon freshly ground black
   pepper
Pinch dried thyme
Pinch dried basil
1 pound Slow-Cooked Venison
   (page 145)
1 (16-ounce) package Cascadian
   Farm frozen Organic Hash
   Browns, thawed
1 (10-ounce) Cascadian Farm
   Organic frozen Gardener's Blend
   Vegetables, thawed
Optional: Fresh parsley sprigs

1. Heat the olive oil and butter in a large, deep nonstick sauté pan. Add the onion and sauté until transparent; stir in the tomato purée and sauté for 2 minutes. Add the garlic and sauté for 1 minute. Add the beef base; stir to dissolve and mix it with the other ingredients.

2. In a mixing cup, whisk together the wine, jelly, water, lemon juice, and cornstarch. Add to the pan and bring to a boil. Add the sugar (if using), parsley, chili powder, mustard powder, pepper, thyme, basil, venison, hash browns, and vegetables; stir to coat. Reduce heat, cover, and simmer for 30 minutes. (Simmer for 45 minutes to 1 hour if the hash browns and vegetables are still frozen when added to the pan.) Serve immediately, garnished with fresh parsley, if desired.

Pork Loin Dinner in Adobo Sauce

1 large sweet onion, thinly sliced

2 tart apples, peeled, cored, and thinly sliced

4 medium-size potatoes, peeled and thinly sliced

1 tablespoon apple cider vinegar

4 teaspoons unsalted butter

4 (5-ounce) pork medallions, cut from boneless loin

2 teaspoons olive or peanut oil

½ teaspoon freshly ground pepper

½ cup Chipotle Peppers in Adobo Sauce (page 252)

¼ teaspoon Minor's Low Sodium Chicken Base

½ cup water

Serves 4	
Per serving:	
Calories:	541.36
Protein:	35.05 g
Carbohydrates:	56.92 g
Total fat:	19.55 g
Sat. fat:	6.44 g
Cholesterol:	105.48 mg
Sodium:	134.76 mg
Fiber:	5.96 g

1. Preheat oven to 200°.
2. In a microwave-safe dish, combine the onion, apples. and potatoes. Top with the vinegar and butter. Cover and microwave on high for 5 minutes or until tender. Leave covered and allow the mixture to "steam" while preparing the pork medallions.
3. Pat the pork medallions dry with paper towels. Rub the oil onto the pork and season with the pepper. Bring a sauté pan treated with nonstick spray to temperature over medium heat. When hot, add the pork and sauté for 3 minutes on each side. Remove the pork from the pan, set the pan aside, and place the meat on a baking sheet in the preheated oven.
4. Once the pork is moved to the warm oven, remove the lid to the potato mixture and test for doneness. Microwave on high for another 2 minutes, if necessary, or until the onion is transparent and the apples and potatoes are tender.
5. Pour off the oil from the sauté pan used for the pork and add the Chipotle Peppers in Adobo Sauce. Over high heat, bring the sauce to a boil while stirring. Stir in the chicken base and stir until dissolved. Add the water and, while continuing to stir, cook over a high heat for 2 to 3 minutes or until the sauce is thick enough to coat the back of a spoon. Set aside and keep warm.
6. Spoon the apples, onion, and potatoes onto the centers of 4 serving plates. Place the sautéed pork medallions atop each and evenly divide the sauce over each serving. Serve immediately.

Italian Spinach and Noodle Casserole

Serves 4	
Per serving:	
Calories:	398.19
Protein:	29.17 g
Carbohydrates:	58.78 g
Total fat:	6.09 g
Sat. fat:	1.93 g
Cholesterol:	125.17 mg
Sodium:	237.90 mg
Fiber:	7.71 g

Spectrum Naturals Extra-Virgin Olive Spray Oil
4 cups cooked no-salt-added oat bran pasta
1 tablespoon lemon juice
1 (10-ounce) package frozen no-salt-added chopped spinach, thawed and squeezed dry
1 cup nonfat cottage cheese
2 large eggs, beaten
⅛ teaspoon freshly grated nutmeg
8 teaspoons grated Parmesan cheese, divided
¼ pound Easy Italian-Seasoned Turkey Sausage (page 134)
2 cups fresh button mushrooms, sliced
2 cups Low-Fat Tomato Sauce (page 199)
Freshly ground black pepper

1. Preheat oven to 350°. Treat an 8" square baking pan with the olive oil spray.
2. Prepare the noodles according to the package directions, except omit salt from the water and add the lemon juice; drain. Set aside and keep warm.
3. Combine the spinach, cottage cheese, eggs, nutmeg, and 4 teaspoons of the Parmesan cheese in a small bowl and mix well.
4. Bring a large, deep nonstick sauté pan treated with the spray oil to temperature over medium heat. Add the turkey sausage; sauté until almost done. Add the mushrooms and sauté for 3 to 5 minutes. Stir in the tomato sauce and bring to temperature.
5. Spoon some of the sauce into the bottom of the prepared baking pan. Arrange half of the pasta over the top of the sauce. Spoon the spinach mixture over the pasta in the baking pan. Cover with a little more of the sauce. Add the remaining pasta to the top of the spinach mixture and sauce. Pour the remaining sauce over the pasta in the baking pan. Sprinkle the remaining 4 teaspoons of Parmesan cheese over the top, and black pepper to taste.
6. Bake for 30 minutes or until casserole is well-heated all the way through and the sauce is bubbling on top. Remove from the oven and let rest for 5 or 10 minutes, then slice and serve with a tossed salad.

New England Boiled Dinner

2 pounds corned beef brisket
1 bay leaf
3 large potatoes, peeled and diced
6 carrots, peeled and sliced
3 large turnips, peeled and diced
4 small sweet or white onions,
    quartered
¼ cup maple syrup
¼ teaspoon mustard powder
1 teaspoon lemon juice
Freshly ground black pepper
Optional: Fresh parsley

Serves 8	
Per serving:	
Calories:	395.08
Protein:	20.00 g
Carbohydrates:	40.40 g
Total fat:	17.22 g
Sat. fat:	5.43 g
Cholesterol:	61.24 mg
Sodium:	214.56 mg
Fiber:	4.84 g

1. Rinse the corned beef in cold water. Place the meat in a large Dutch oven treated with nonstick spray. Cover with water. Add the bay leaf. Bring to a boil over medium-high heat; reduce heat and simmer, covered, for 1½ hours.

2. Preheat oven to 400°. Add the potatoes, carrots, turnips, and onions to a saucepan and cover with cold water. Bring to a boil over medium-high heat; reduce heat, cover, and simmer for 30 minutes or until tender.

3. Once the vegetables are cooking, remove the meat from the Dutch oven and discard the broth and bay leaf. Place the boiled meat in a roasting pan treated with nonstick spray. In a small bowl, combine the maple syrup with the mustard powder and lemon juice. Drizzle the maple syrup mixture over the meat. Bake, uncovered, for 20 minutes. Remove to a serving platter, tent with aluminum foil, and let stand for 10 minutes.

4. Ladle about ½ cup of the vegetable water into the roasting pan and scrape the bottom of the pan to incorporate the water into the drippings. Remove the boiled vegetables from the saucepan with a slotted spoon and place in the roasting pan; toss with the juices. Place in the oven while the meat rests.

5. Slice the brisket thinly across the grain. Fan out on the serving platter. Remove the vegetables from the oven and arrange them around the brisket. Sprinkle with freshly ground black pepper to taste. Garnish with fresh parsley, if desired. Serve immediately.

Beef Barbecue

Serves 6	
Per serving:	
Calories:	290.81
Protein:	40.77 g
Carbohydrates:	8.49 g
Total fat:	8.17 g
Sat. fat:	2.89 g
Cholesterol:	102.00 mg
Sodium:	92.97 mg
Fiber:	0.26 g

1½ pounds Easy Slow-Cooked
 "Roast" Beef (page 145)
1 cup water
½ cup dry white wine
½ cup low-salt ketchup
1 tablespoon red wine vinegar
2 teaspoons Lea & Perrins
 Worcestershire sauce

2 teaspoons mustard powder
1 tablespoon dried minced onion
1 teaspoon dried minced garlic
1 teaspoon cracked black pepper
1 tablespoon brown sugar
¼ teaspoon salt-free chili powder
Pinch dried red pepper flakes,
 crushed

1. Add the cooked beef to the slow cooker. Mix together all the remaining ingredients and pour over the beef. Add additional water, to cover the meat. Set the slow cooker on high until the mixture begins to boil.
2. Reduce heat to low and simmer for 2 or more hours, until tender. Adjust the seasonings, if necessary.

Slow-Cooked Hearty Beef and Cabbage Soup

Serves 4	
Per serving:	
Calories:	238.20
Protein:	20.29 g
Carbohydrates:	29.88 g
Total fat:	4.39 g
Sat. fat:	1.35 g
Cholesterol:	38.66 mg
Sodium:	200.92 mg
Fiber:	6.96 g

¼ pound Easy Slow-Cooked
 "Roast" Beef (page 145)
1 small head of cabbage, chopped
1 medium-size white or yellow
 onion, chopped
2 carrots, thinly sliced
¼ cup uncooked long-grain brown
 rice
2 stalks celery, sliced into ½" pieces

1 clove garlic, minced
3 cups nonfat, low-salt beef broth
2 (14.5-ounce) cans Muir Glen
 Organic No Salt Added Diced
 Tomatoes
½ cup water
¼ teaspoon granulated sugar
⅛ teaspoon freshly ground black
 pepper

Add the cooked beef to the slow cooker. Mix together all the remaining ingredients and pour over the beef. Set the slow cooker on high until the mixture begins to boil. Reduce heat to low and simmer for 8 to 10 hours. Adjust seasonings, if necessary.

Easy Chicken Barbecue

Serves 4	
Per serving:	
Calories:	211.30
Protein:	35.49 g
Carbohydrates:	5.50 g
Total fat:	4.15 g
Sat. fat:	1.17 g
Cholesterol:	96.40 mg
Sodium:	106.98 mg
Fiber:	0.23 g

1 tablespoon water or chicken
   broth or lemon juice
1 small sweet onion, chopped
1 clove garlic, chopped

1 pound Easy Slow-Cooked
   Chicken
¼ cup Mr. Spice Honey Barbecue
   Sauce

1. In a medium-size microwave-safe bowl, combine the water, onion, and garlic; microwave on high for 3 minutes or until the onion is transparent.
2. Add the chicken and barbecue sauce to the bowl; mix well. Cover and microwave at 70 percent power for 2 minutes or until the chicken is heated through; stir and serve.

Easy Slow-Cooked Chicken

Serves 8	
Per serving:	
Calories:	47.22
Protein:	8.81 g
Carbohydrates:	0.07 g
Total fat:	1.03 g
Sat. fat:	0.29 g
Cholesterol:	24.12 mg
Sodium:	26.60 mg
Fiber:	0.00 g

1½ pounds bone-in chicken pieces
½ teaspoon Minor's Low Sodium
   Chicken Base
⅛ teaspoon Minor's Roasted
   Mirepoix Flavor Concentrate

Optional: ½ teaspoon dried minced
   onion
Optional: ¼ teaspoon dried minced
   garlic
Water, as needed

1. Put all the ingredients in a ceramic-lined slow cooker, adding enough water to cover the chicken; set the cooker on high. Once the mixture begins to boil, stir to dissolve the bases; reduce temperature to low. Simmer for 8 or more hours, until tender.
2. Remove the chicken from the slow cooker and discard the broth (or refrigerate the broth for a later use). Separate the meat from the bone; discard the skin, fat, and bones. Weigh the meat and separate it into 1-ounce servings. The meat can be kept for 1 or 2 days in the refrigerator, or freeze portions for use later.

Easy Ginger Cashew Chicken and Broccoli

Serves 4	
Per serving:	
Calories:	286.88
Protein:	38.89 g
Carbohydrates:	14.23 g
Total fat:	8.38 g
Sat. fat:	2.01 g
Cholesterol:	96.48 mg
Sodium:	127.39 mg
Fiber:	0.47 g

1 tablespoon water or chicken
  broth or lemon juice
1 small sweet onion, chopped
1 clove garlic, chopped
4 cups broccoli florets
1 pound cooked dark meat chicken

6 tablespoons Mr. Spice Ginger
  Stir-Fry Sauce
¼ cup unsalted dry-roasted cashew
  pieces
Optional: Candied ginger, minced

In a large microwave-safe bowl, combine the water, onion, garlic, and broccoli. Cover and microwave on high for 4 minutes or until the broccoli is crisp-tender. Add the chicken and stir-fry sauce; stir well. Microwave at 70 percent power for 2 minutes or until the mixture is heated through. Serve over cooked rice; top each serving with 1 table-spoon of the cashews, and minced candied ginger, if desired.

Easy Slow-Cooked Pork

Serves 12	
Per serving:	
Calories:	372.05
Protein:	26.53 g
Carbohydrates:	0.04 g
Total fat:	28.73 g
Sat. fat:	10.44 g
Cholesterol:	104.30 mg
Sodium:	76.94 mg
Fiber:	0.00 g

4½-pound bone-in lean pork roast
1 teaspoon Minor's Pork Base, no MSG
¼ teaspoon Minor's Roasted
  Mirepoix Flavor Concentrate

1 tablespoon dried minced onion
1 teaspoon dried minced garlic
Water, as needed

1. Put the roast and all the other ingredients in a ceramic-lined slow cooker, adding enough water to cover the roast; set the cooker on high. Once the mixture begins to boil, stir to dissolve the bases; reduce temperature to low. Allow the meat to simmer for 8 or more hours, until tender.
2. Separate the meat from the resulting broth; discard the broth (or refrigerate it for a later use). Remove any remaining fat from the meat and take the meat off the bone; discard the fat and bone. Weigh the meat and separate it into 4-ounce servings. The meat can be kept for 1 or 2 days in the refrigerator, or freeze portions for use later.

Pepped-Up Pork Sandwiches

1 large white or yellow onion, chopped

1 large red bell pepper, seeded and chopped

1 large green bell pepper, seeded and chopped

1 clove garlic, minced

3 tablespoons pork broth

1 tablespoon Mr. Spice Garlic Steak Sauce

½ pound cooked pork, shredded

8 slices, thinly sliced low-salt bread

Serves 4	
Per serving:	
Calories:	320.40
Protein:	17.44 g
Carbohydrates:	25.57 g
Total fat:	16.17 g
Sat. fat:	5.65 g
Cholesterol:	53.48 mg
Sodium:	109.68 mg
Fiber:	1.59 g

In a medium-size microwave-safe bowl, combine the onion, peppers, garlic, and broth; microwave on high for 5 minutes or until the onion is transparent and the peppers are soft. Add the steak sauce and pork; stir to combine. Cover and microwave at 70 percent power for 2 minutes or until the mixture is heated through. Taste and add more steak sauce, if desired. Serve immediately, as sandwiches on plain or toasted bread.

Easy Sweet-and-Sour Pork

1 large white or yellow onion, cut into large dice

1 large green bell pepper, seeded and chopped

1 clove garlic, minced

⅛ cup (2 tablespoons) dry sherry or pork broth or water

½ pound cooked pork, shredded

¼ cup Mr. Spice Sweet & Sour Sauce

Serves 4	
Per serving:	
Calories:	228.64
Protein:	14.11 g
Carbohydrates:	10.25 g
Total fat:	14.54 g
Sat. fat:	5.25 g
Cholesterol:	52.24 mg
Sodium:	85.93 mg
Fiber:	1.19 g

In a medium-size microwave-safe bowl, combine the onion, pepper, garlic, and sherry; microwave on high for 3 minutes or until the vegetables are crisp-tender. Add the sweet-and-sour sauce and pork; stir to combine. Cover and microwave at 70 percent power for 2 minutes or until the mixture is heated through. Taste and add more sweet-and-sour sauce, if desired.

Warm Pork Salad

Serves 2	
Per serving:	
Calories:	255.00
Protein:	14.37 g
Carbohydrates:	16.52 g
Total fat:	14.80 g
Sat. fat:	5.28 g
Cholesterol:	52.00 mg
Sodium:	51.52 mg
Fiber:	3.29 g

¼ pound Easy Slow-Cooked Pork (page 152)
2 tablespoons Mr. Spice Honey Mustard Sauce
1 Granny Smith or Golden Delicious apple, sliced

2 slices red onion
2 cups coleslaw mix
4 drops toasted sesame oil
Dash freshly ground black pepper

1. In a small nonstick sauté pan treated with nonstick spray, stir-fry the leftover pork until warm. Add the honey mustard sauce; mix until well-blended.
2. Add the apple, onion, and coleslaw mix; stir, then cover and cook for 2 minutes or until the vegetables are crisp-tender.
3. Top the salads with 2 drops each of the sesame oil and some freshly ground black pepper.

Pork Barbecue Sandwiches

Serves 4	
Per serving:	
Calories:	415.31
Protein:	18.06 g
Carbohydrates:	43.15 g
Total fat:	19.22 g
Sat. fat:	6.38 g
Cholesterol:	52.00 mg
Sodium:	100.75 mg
Fiber:	3.71 g

Spectrum Naturals Canola Spray Oil
2 teaspoons canola oil
1 small Granny Smith or Golden Delicious apple, peeled, cored, and grated
1 small sweet onion, finely minced
2 tablespoons Mr. Spice Honey Mustard Sauce

2 tablespoons Mr. Spice Honey Barbecue Sauce
⅛ teaspoon freshly ground black pepper
½ pound Easy Slow-Cooked Pork (page 152)
8 (1-ounce) slices Old-Style Whole-Wheat Bread (page 215)

Bring a nonstick sauté pan treated with spray oil to temperature over medium heat. Add the oil, apple, and onion; sauté until the onion is transparent. Add the sauces and pepper; mix well. Add the pork and simmer with the sauces, stirring until heated through. Evenly divide the pork mixture over 4 slices of the bread; top with the remaining 4 slices. Serve immediately.

Baked Pork Tenderloin Dinner

4 small Yukon gold potatoes,
   scrubbed, peeled, and sliced
4 (2-ounce) pieces trimmed boneless pork loin, pounded flat
4 Granny Smith or Golden
   Delicious apples, peeled, cored,
   and sliced
1 large sweet onion, sliced

1 tablespoon minced shallots
⅛ cup apple cider or apple juice
⅛ teaspoon mustard powder
⅛ teaspoon dried lemon granules,
   crushed
⅛ teaspoon freshly ground black
   pepper

Serves 4	
Per serving:	
Calories:	262.26
Protein:	13.44 g
Carbohydrates:	36.26 g
Total fat:	7.73 g
Sat. fat:	2.59 g
Cholesterol:	37.99 mg
Sodium:	48.37 mg
Fiber:	4.77 g

1. Preheat oven to 350°. Treat an ovenproof casserole dish with nonstick spray.
2. Layer the potato slices from 2 of the potatoes across the bottom of the prepared dish. Top with 2 pieces of the flattened pork loin. Arrange the apple and onion slices over the top of the loin. Sprinkle the shallots over the apples and onion. Top with the remaining flattened pork loins.
3. In a small bowl or measuring cup, mix together the apple cider (or juice), mustard powder, lemon granules, and pepper. Drizzle the apple cider mixture over the top of the casserole. Cover and bake for 45 minutes or until the potatoes and apples are tender. Leave the casserole covered and let rest for 10 minutes after you remove it from the oven.

Salmon Scramble

Serves 4	
Per serving:	
Calories:	215.50
Protein:	17.76 g
Carbohydrates:	18.58 g
Total fat:	8.53 g
Sat. fat:	2.23 g
Cholesterol:	225.60 mg
Sodium:	289.66 mg
Fiber:	5.14 g

4 cups chopped broccoli (fresh or frozen)

2 (1-ounce) slices French Bread (page 216)

4 large eggs

2 teaspoons Hellmann's or Best Foods Real Mayonnaise

1 teaspoon Cascadian Farm Sweet Relish

¼ teaspoon mustard powder

⅛ teaspoon dried lemon granules, crushed

½ teaspoon Fines Herbes (page 276) or Herbes de Provence (page 276)

1 tablespoon yellow cornmeal

4 ounces canned salmon, drained

1. In a microwave-safe covered bowl, steam the broccoli for 5 minutes or until tender. Drain off any moisture from the broccoli; add the broccoli to a large, deep nonstick sauté pan treated with nonstick spray and dry-sauté over medium heat to remove any excess moisture.
2. Put the French Bread in a blender or food processor; process to make bread crumbs.
3. In a bowl, beat together the eggs, mayonnaise, relish, mustard powder, lemon granules, and herbs. Fold in the cornmeal, salmon, and bread crumbs. Pour the salmon mixture over the broccoli and toss to mix. Cook until the eggs are done, stirring the mixture occasionally with a spatula.

❋ Freezing Meat

Most cooked meats wrapped in foil or placed in sealable plastic freezer bags can be stored in the freezer for 3 months, or up to 2 years if frozen in vacuum-sealed plastic containers.

Baked Cauliflower Casserole

1¾-pound head cauliflower
1 teaspoon lemon juice
⅛ teaspoon mustard powder
Spectrum Naturals Canola Spray
   Oil with Butter Flavor
2 large eggs, beaten

1 teaspoon Sonoran Spice Blend
  (see page 275)
¼ cup grated Parmesan cheese
½ cup bread crumbs

Serves 6	
Per serving:	
Calories:	84.73
Protein:	6.57 g
Carbohydrates:	7.77 g
Total fat:	3.66 g
Sat. fat:	1.42 g
Cholesterol:	74.16 mg
Sodium:	139.16 mg
Fiber:	3.66 g

1. Preheat oven to 375°.
2. Trim off the outer leaves of the cauliflower. Break the cauliflower apart. Bring a large pot of water to boil over medium-high heat. Add the lemon juice and mustard powder; stir to mix. Add the cauliflower to the water and blanch for 5 minutes. Remove with a slotted spoon and drain.
3. Treat a ovenproof casserole dish with the spray oil. Spread the cauliflower evenly in the casserole dish.
4. In a small bowl, mix together the eggs, spice blend, and cheese. Evenly pour the mixture over the top of the cauliflower. Sprinkle the bread crumbs over the top and lightly mist with the spray oil. Cover and bake for 15 minutes or until the eggs are set and the cheese is melted.

❁ Crunchier Bread Crumbs

To further crisp the bread crumbs that top the Baked Cauliflower Casserole, remove the cover once the casserole is baked and mist again with additional spray oil; then, either return the casserole to the oven for an additional 5 to 10 minutes or place under the broiler until the bread crumbs are lightly browned.

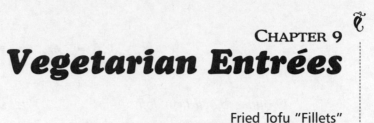

CHAPTER 9

Vegetarian Entrées

Fried Tofu "Fillets"

Serves 4	
Per serving:	
Calories:	155.79
Protein:	12.72 g
Carbohydrates:	7.28 g
Total fat:	9.46 g
Sat. fat:	1.54 g
Cholesterol:	46.75 mg
Sodium:	58.44 mg
Fiber:	0.73 g

19-ounce block firm tofu
¼ cup nonfat, low-sodium chicken-
   flavored broth
¼ teaspoon Worcestershire sauce
¼ teaspoon Bragg Liquid Aminos
Optional: A few dashes of hot
   pepper sauce
1 tablespoon water
1 tablespoon unbleached all-purpose flour
2 teaspoons masa harina or cornmeal

1 teaspoon white rice flour
¼ teaspoon dried basil
¼ teaspoon dried rosemary
Pinch dried sage
Pinch dried marjoram
Pinch dried thyme
Pinch dried oregano
1 egg
2 teaspoons olive or canola oil

1. Slice the tofu into 4 equal pieces. Place the slices between layers of
   paper towels and fold the towels over in both directions to cover the
   tofu. Place a baking sheet on top of the tofu and weigh it down with
   a cast iron skillet or similar weight for 1 hour.
2. In a casserole dish wide enough to hold the tofu slices side by side,
   combine the broth, Worcestershire sauce, Bragg Liquid Aminos, hot
   pepper sauce (if using), and water. Place the tofu into the broth marinade; marinate for 15 minutes on each side.
3. Place the flour, masa (or cornmeal), and rice flour into a shallow
   dish and mix until combined. Mix together the dried basil, rosemary,
   sage, marjoram, thyme, and oregano; grind using a spice grinder or a
   mortar and pestle, then add to the flour mixture and mix well. In a
   small bowl, beat the egg until frothy.
4. Heat the oil in a nonstick skillet over medium-high heat.
5. Remove the tofu from the broth marinade and drain on paper towels
   to remove any excess marinade. Lightly dredge the tofu in the flour
   mixture, knocking off any excess flour. Dip the floured slices into the
   egg until completely, but thinly, coated on both sides.
6. Gently place the tofu in the skillet and fry for 2 minutes per side, until
   golden brown.

Pasta in Mushroom Alfredo-Style Sauce

1 teaspoon extra-virgin olive oil
1 teaspoon unsalted butter
2 cups sliced button or cremini
  mushrooms
1 small onion, minced
4 cloves garlic, minced
2 teaspoons unbleached all-purpose
  flour
½ teaspoon basil or an herb seasoning blend
¼ teaspoon freshly ground black
  pepper

2 pinches dried red pepper flakes
Pinch ground nutmeg
⅛ cup skim milk
2 cups nonfat cottage cheese
¼ cup grated Parmesan cheese
8 ounces dry oat bran or whole-
  wheat pasta
2 tablespoons fresh lemon juice
1 teaspoon dried parsley
Optional: 4 teaspoons chopped
  unsalted, dry-roasted peanuts

Serves 4	
Per serving:	
Calories:	343.04
Protein:	25.49 g
Carbohydrates:	50.69 g
Total fat:	5.31 g
Sat. fat:	2.33 g
Cholesterol:	12.99 mg
Sodium:	144.34 mg
Fiber:	1.16 g

1. In a deep nonstick skillet, heat the olive oil and butter over medium-high heat. Add the mushrooms and sauté for 2 minutes. Add the onion and garlic; sauté for 2 minutes or until the onion is transparent. Stir often to prevent the garlic from burning.

2. Sprinkle the flour over the mushroom mixture. Cook for 1 minute, stirring well so the flour absorbs any liquid and oil and makes a light roux. Add the basil, pepper, 1 dash of the red pepper flakes, and the nutmeg; stir to combine.

3. Add the milk and stir to loosen the roux. Add the cottage cheese. (For a smoother sauce, purée the cottage cheese in a blender or food processor before adding it to the pan.) Cook and stir until the sauce is thickened and smooth. Add all but 4 teaspoons of the grated Parmesan cheese and stir well.

4. Lower the heat and keep the sauce warm while the pasta cooks. Consult the package directions for the amount of water and cooking time for the pasta. Add the lemon juice and the remaining dash of red pepper flakes to the boiling water, then add the pasta. Cook until al dente, then drain well. Toss the drained pasta with the sauce. Sprinkle with the parsley and the reserved Parmesan cheese. Top each serving with 1 teaspoon chopped peanuts, if desired.

Walnut and Mushroom Loaf

Serves 4	
Per serving:	
Calories:	786.26
Protein:	26.49 g
Carbohydrates:	57.98 g
Total fat:	48.92 g
Sat. fat:	5.03 g
Cholesterol:	0.00 mg
Sodium:	243.25 mg
Fiber:	13.73 g

5 teaspoons walnut or olive oil
1 large sweet onion, chopped
4 cups button mushrooms, sliced
1 cup ground walnuts
1 cup ground raw sunflower seeds
1 tablespoon lemon juice
1⅓ cups soymilk
1 cup whole-wheat bread crumbs
½ teaspoon dried parsley
⅛ teaspoon dried sage
1 teaspoon dried basil
½ cup oatmeal
1⅓ cups warm water
1 tablespoon yeast extract
(such as Marmite)

1. Preheat oven to 350°. Treat a baking dish with nonstick spray.
2. Bring a large nonstick sauté pan treated with nonstick spray to temperature over medium heat. Add 4 teaspoons of the oil, the onion, and mushrooms; sauté for 3 minutes. Add the walnuts and sunflower seeds; stir to mix, and sauté for 1 minute. Remove the pan from the heat and stir in the lemon juice, soymilk, bread crumbs, parsley, sage, and basil. Transfer to the prepared baking dish; bake for 45 minutes.
3. While the loaf bakes, prepare the gravy by putting the oatmeal, water, and the remaining 1 teaspoon oil in the bowl of a blender or food processor; pulse until liquefied. Pour the mixture into a small nonstick saucepan and heat over medium-low heat, stirring constantly until thickened. Stir in the yeast extract. Serve warm over the loaf.

❀ Be Creative
You can substitute steamed vegetables like carrots and some cooked beans for some of the mushrooms in the Walnut and Mushroom Loaf. Likewise, experiment using your favorite seasoning blends instead of the recommended dried herbs.

Cashew Corn Chowder

4 teaspoons canola oil
1 large sweet onion, chopped
4 stalks celery, chopped
1 medium-size sweet potato,
    peeled and diced
3 cloves garlic, minced
1 tablespoon unbleached all-pur-
    pose flour
6 cups water
1 (10-ounce) package Cascadian
    Farm frozen Organic Super
    Sweet Corn, thawed

1 small red bell pepper, seeded
    and diced
1 small green bell pepper, seeded
    and diced
½ cup no-salt-added roasted
    cashew butter
1 tablespoon fresh lime juice
1 teaspoon dried cilantro, crushed
1/16 teaspoon cayenne
⅛ teaspoon freshly ground black
    pepper

Serves 4	
Per serving:	
Calories:	357.65
Protein:	9.72 g
Carbohydrates:	40.42 g
Total fat:	21.00 g
Sat. fat:	3.49 g
Cholesterol:	0.00 mg
Sodium:	36.25 mg
Fiber:	4.21 g

1. Heat the oil in a large saucepan on medium-high. Add the onions and celery; sauté for 3 to 4 minutes, stirring frequently. Add the sweet potatoes; sauté for 1 or 2 minutes, mixing them in with the other vegetables. Add the garlic and sauté for 1 minute.
2. Lower the heat to medium and stir in the flour. Continue to stir for 5 minutes to completely cook the flour. Add the water and bring to a boil; reduce the heat, cover the pot, and simmer for 40 minutes or until the sweet potatoes are completely tender. Stir well, mashing the sweet potatoes somewhat with the back of a spoon or use a hand blender to cream the soup.
3. Stir in the corn. Return the cover to the pan and simmer for 20 more minutes.
4. Add the bell peppers; cover and simmer for 5 minutes. Add the cashew butter, stirring to blend it completely. Stir in the lime juice, cilantro, cayenne, and pepper. Serve warm.

Mushroom Broth

Serves 8	
Per serving:	
Calories:	20.00
Protein:	3.00 g
Carbohydrates:	0.00 g
Total fat:	0.00 g
Sat. fat:	0.00 g
Cholesterol:	0.00 mg
Sodium:	35.00 mg
Fiber:	0.00 g

4 carrots, washed and cut into large pieces
2 large leeks, well-cleaned and cut into large pieces
2 large sweet onions, quartered
1 stalk celery, chopped
5 whole cloves
Pinch dried red pepper flakes
2 cups sliced fresh button or other fresh mushrooms
9 cups water

Put all the ingredients in a large pot and bring to a boil; reduce heat and simmer, covered, for 45 minutes. Strain the broth for a clear stock. Can be refrigerated for 2 or 3 days, or frozen for 3 months.

Whole-Wheat Pasta in Tomato Butter

Serves 4	
Per serving:	
Calories:	293.12
Protein:	10.27 g
Carbohydrates:	40.73 g
Total fat:	11.03 g
Sat. fat:	6.82 g
Cholesterol:	27.95 mg
Sodium:	166.71 mg
Fiber:	6.70 g

4 cups cooked whole-wheat pasta (no salt added; boiled in lemon juice-seasoned water)
½ cup Tomato Butter (page 249)
4 tablespoons chopped fresh basil
¼ teaspoon freshly ground black pepper
4 tablespoons freshly grated Parmesan cheese

In a large bowl, toss the cooked, drained pasta with the tomato butter, basil, and pepper. Divide among 4 serving plates and top each serving with 1 tablespoon of the Parmesan cheese. Serve immediately.

Black Bean Chili

1½ cups dried black beans
2 tablespoons canola oil
2 large sweet onions, chopped
5 medium-size cloves garlic,
    minced
1 tablespoon ground cumin
1 tablespoon dried oregano
3 tablespoons salt-free chili powder
1 teaspoon freshly ground black
    pepper
1 teaspoon dried red peppers flakes
1 teaspoon dried lemon granules,
    crushed
3 jalapeño peppers, seeded and
    minced

2 (14½-ounce) cans Muir Glen
    Organic No Salt Added Diced
    Tomatoes
1 cup chopped fresh pineapple
4 large carrots, peeled and sliced
1 cup uncooked long-grain brown
    rice
1 tablespoon apple cider or red
    wine vinegar
Optional: Tamari sauce or Bragg
    Liquid Aminos
Optional: No-salt-added peanut
    butter or other nut butter
Fresh cilantro, for garnish

Serves 8	
Per serving:	
Calories:	304.06
Protein:	11.59 g
Carbohydrates:	55.03 g
Total fat:	4.85 g
Sat. fat:	0.61 g
Cholesterol:	0.00 mg
Sodium:	54.88 mg
Fiber:	9.11 g

1. Rinse the beans and cover them with water in a large, heavy pot. Bring to a full boil over medium-high heat, drain, and rinse again. Return the beans to the pot over medium-high heat and add 7 cups of water, or a combination of water and mushroom broth. Once the water comes to a boil, reduce heat and simmer for 1 hour.

2. While the beans cook, bring a large nonstick sauté pan to temperature over medium heat. Add the oil and onions; sauté for 4 minutes, stirring frequently. Lower the heat to medium-low. Add the garlic and sauté for 1 minute. Stir in the cumin, oregano, chili powder, pepper, red pepper flakes, lemon granules, and jalapeños; sauté for an additional 4 minutes, then add the tomatoes. Simmer for 10 minutes, stirring frequently.

3. Stir the sautéed mixture into the pot of beans. Add the pineapple, carrots, and rice. Simmer partially covered for another hour, or until the beans are soft and the rice is done. Stir in the vinegar. Have tamari sauce or Bragg Liquid Aminos, peanut or other nut butter, and freshly ground black pepper available at the table to flavor individual servings of the chili, if desired. Garnish with cilantro.

Spanakopita

Serves 20 (3 triangles per serving)	
Per serving:	
Calories:	120.00
Protein:	5.00 g
Carbohydrates:	18.00 g
Total fat:	3.50 g
Sat. fat:	0.00 g
Cholesterol:	0.00 mg
Sodium:	230.00 mg
Fiber:	0.00 g

½ teaspoon extra-virgin olive oil
1 large sweet onion, chopped
4 cloves garlic, minced
2 cups chopped button mushrooms
1 cup chopped fresh shiitake
  mushrooms
¼ cup dry white wine
5 packed cups chopped spinach
1¼ cups crumbled extra-firm tofu
2 teaspoons dried oregano
2 teaspoons dried basil

2 teaspoons dried parsley
2 teaspoons miso paste
1 teaspoon tamari or soy sauce
½ teaspoon freshly ground black
  pepper
⅛ teaspoon ground nutmeg
1 (16-ounce) package phyllo dough
Spectrum Naturals Extra-Virgin
  Olive Spray Oil

1. Preheat oven to 350°. Line a baking sheet with parchment paper.
2. To prepare the filling, heat a nonstick sauté pan over medium-high heat. Add the olive oil. Add the onion and sauté for 2 minutes or until transparent. Add the garlic and sauté for 1 minute. Add the mushrooms and cook for 1 more minute. Pour in the wine, bring to a boil, and cook until the pan is almost dry, about 2 minutes. Add the spinach and toss with the onion-mushroom mixture, cooking until just wilted, about 2 minutes. Remove from the pan and let cool completely.
3. In a mixing bowl, combine the cooled sautéed vegetables, tofu, herbs, miso, tamari, pepper, and nutmeg; mix well and set aside.
4. Lay out the phyllo dough on a baking sheet and cover with a damp cloth. On a cutting board, lay out 1 sheet of phyllo. Lightly mist the phyllo sheet with olive oil spray. Repeat to make a total of 3 layers.
5. Cut the sheet of phyllo vertically into 6 strips. Place 1 tablespoon of the spinach mixture on the end of each phyllo strip. Fold the bottom left corner to the right top corner, over the spinach mixture. Continue to fold about 4 times to completely seal, creating a small triangle. Place the triangles on the prepared baking sheet. Lightly mist the top of the triangles with the spray oil. Keep covered with damp towel until all the triangles are made. Bake for 15 to 20 minutes or until golden brown.

Mushroom Risotto

2 tablespoons olive oil
4 cloves garlic, minced
1 tablespoon minced shallots
2 cups uncooked brown arborio
  or basmati rice
½ cup dry white wine
2 cups Mushroom Broth (page 164)

1–2 cups boiling water
2 tablespoons unsalted butter
⅛ teaspoon ground mustard
Pinch cayenne pepper
2 tablespoons grated Parmesan
  cheese

Serves 8	
Per serving:	
Calories:	260.44
Protein:	4.73 g
Carbohydrates:	38.99 g
Total fat:	8.06 g
Sat. fat:	2.77 g
Cholesterol:	8.76 mg
Sodium:	35.06 mg
Fiber:	2.17 g

1. Bring a large, deep nonstick sauté pan to temperature over medium heat; add the olive oil, garlic, and shallots; sauté for 1 minute, being careful not to burn the garlic. Add the rice and stir to coat it with the olive oil. Add the wine and bring to a simmer, reducing the heat, if necessary, to maintain a simmer.

2. Pour the mushroom broth and 1 cup of the water into a saucepan over medium heat; once it comes to temperature, adjust the heat to maintain a simmer.

3. Ladle about ½ cup of the warm mushroom broth into the rice. At this point, begin stirring the rice constantly, adding more broth ½ cup at a time once the broth is absorbed into the rice. Continue to cook until the rice is al dente, using the additional cup of water, if necessary. The entire cooking process should take about 20 to 25 minutes.

4. Lower the heat. Add the butter, ground mustard, cayenne, and Parmesan cheese; stir rapidly to combine and melt the butter and cheese into the risotto. The rice is ready when it retains a thick, creamy consistency.

❀ Nonstick Spray

You can make your own nonstick spray by adding ¼ cup liquid lecithin and ¾ cup of your choice of oil to a mister or pump spray bottle. Mix or shake well before each use.

Tomato and Vegetable Frittata

Serves 4	
Per serving:	
Calories:	184.02
Protein:	10.36 g
Carbohydrates:	10.93 g
Total fat:	11.43 g
Sat. fat:	4.30 g
Cholesterol:	222.62 mg
Sodium:	211.46 mg
Fiber:	2.39 g

1 cup grated zucchini, seeded
2 cups cherry tomatoes
Spectrum Naturals Extra-Virgin
*   Olive Spray Oil or other non-*
*   stick spray*
2 teaspoons olive oil
2 teaspoons unsalted butter, melted
*   and cooled*
1 stalk celery, finely minced
2 carrots, peeled and grated
1 large sweet onion, sliced

4 large eggs
½ teaspoon dried basil
¼ teaspoon dried parsley
⅛ teaspoon freshly ground black
*   pepper*
Pinch chili powder
Pinch mustard powder
Pinch dried red pepper flakes
¼ cup grated Parmesan cheese
Optional: Freshly grated nutmeg

1. Place the grated zucchini between several layers of paper towels and squeeze out the water; set aside. Cut the cherry tomatoes in half and return them to the measuring cup; set aside to allow the juices to drain.

2. Treat a large, nonstick, ovenproof sauté pan with a thin coating of the spray oil. Bring to temperature over medium heat. Add the olive oil and butter. When the butter sizzles, add the celery and carrots; sauté for 3 minutes or until almost tender. Pour the accumulated juices from the tomatoes into a measuring cup; set aside. Add the onion, tomatoes, and zucchini; sauté for 5 minutes or until the onion is transparent and additional moisture from the tomatoes and zucchini has evaporated from the pan. (Stir occasionally during the sautéing process to mix the vegetables.)

3. Add enough water to the tomato juices to equal ⅛ cup, if necessary, and whisk together with the eggs; stir in the basil, parsley, pepper, chili powder, mustard powder, and red pepper flakes. Pour the mixture over the sautéed vegetables in the pan. Tilt the pan so that the eggs run around to the edges. Use a spoon or spatula to gently stir the eggs into the vegetables, so that some of the eggs run to the bottom of the pan. Cook the eggs on the stovetop for about 3 minutes, until they just begin to set in the center. (Try to arrange it so that a lot of the tomato halves are at the top of the frittata.)

4. Remove the pan from the burner and sprinkle the Parmesan cheese evenly over the top of the frittata. Place the pan under the broiler for 1 to 2 minutes, until the cheese is melted and lightly browned. Watch carefully to avoid burning the frittata. Gently lift the edges of the frittata away from the pan with a spatula. Jiggle the pan to loosen the frittata, then slide it onto a serving platter. Use a knife or pizza cutter to cut into wedges. Serve with freshly grated nutmeg over the top, if desired.

❀ Sesame Oil

Sesame oil has a low smoke point so it isn't suitable for high-temperature stir-frying. It is also expensive. There are times, however, when the subtle taste it imparts to a dish is worth babying it a bit. You can make a mighty fine substitute by adding ⅛ cup of sesame seeds to a small saucepan over medium heat; dry-toast for about 1 minute or until they just begin to pop and turn color. Add ½ cup of cold-pressed canola or sunflower seed oil and cook for 1 to 2 minutes, until the oil is heated through. Purée in a blender or use a hand blender. Cover and let rest at room temperature for 2 hours; strain out the seeds by pouring the oil through a sieve lined with cheesecloth.

Couscous in Black Olive–Lemon Vinaigrette

Serves 4	
Per serving:	
Calories:	452.67
Protein:	11.14 g
Carbohydrates:	68.16 g
Total fat:	15.48 g
Sat. fat:	2.15 g
Cholesterol:	0.05 mg
Sodium:	177.39 mg
Fiber:	7.03 g

2½ cups water
1⅔ cups couscous
1 teaspoon dried parsley
1 teaspoon dried cilantro
1 teaspoon Minor's Roasted Mirepoix Flavor Concentrate
8 large canned black olives (not in brine), pitted and finely minced
¼ cup extra-virgin olive oil
1 tablespoon fresh lemon juice
⅛ teaspoon freshly ground black pepper
Pinch mustard powder
Pinch ground cumin
Pinch cayenne pepper or dried red pepper flakes
2 medium-size zucchini, seeded and chopped
1 large tomato, peeled, seeded, and chopped
2 stalks celery, chopped
2 carrots, peeled and grated
1 large cucumber, peeled, seeded, and chopped
¼ cup unsalted almonds, coarsely ground and toasted in a dry pan over medium heat

1. Boil the water. In a large bowl, mix together the couscous, parsley, and cilantro. Dissolve the base in the boiling water; pour the boiling mixture over the couscous. Cover and set aside for 10 minutes; once the mixture is absorbed, fluff the couscous with a fork.
2. Rinse the black olives in cold water; pat dry between paper towels. Add the olives to a jar along with the olive oil, lemon juice, pepper, mustard powder, cumin, and cayenne pepper (or red pepper flakes); cover and shake well. Set aside.
3. Add the zucchini, tomato, celery, carrots, cucumber, and almonds to the bowl with the couscous and toss to mix. Shake the jar of vinaigrette until the dressing is emulsified; pour over the couscous and toss.

❁ Egg Substitute
When a recipe like meatloaf calls for egg "to bind the meat and other ingredients," you can use this egg substitute instead: Mix 1 tablespoon of ground flaxseed with ¼ cup water; microwave on high for 15 to 30 seconds, or until it has the consistency of egg whites when stirred.

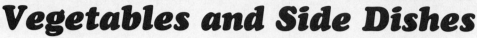

CHAPTER 10 ⁋

Vegetables and Side Dishes

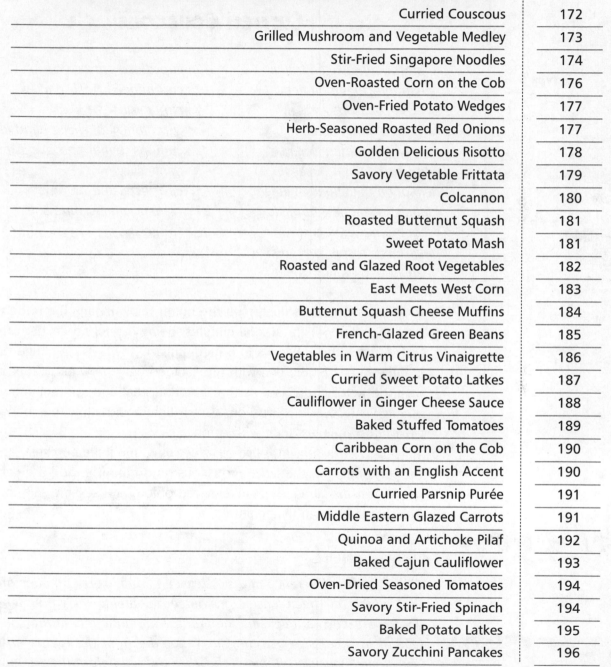

Curried Couscous

Serves 6	
Per serving:	
Calories:	386.42
Protein:	9.75 g
Carbohydrates:	49.04 g
Total fat:	17.76 g
Sat. fat:	3.01 g
Cholesterol:	5.39 mg
Sodium:	84.55 mg
Fiber:	4.82 g

1 tablespoon unsalted butter
1 teaspoon curry powder
1½ cups couscous
1½ cups boiling water
¼ cup plain nonfat yogurt
¼ cup extra-virgin olive oil
1 teaspoon white wine vinegar
¼ teaspoon ground turmeric
¼ teaspoon lemon zest
1 teaspoon freshly ground black
   pepper

½ cup diced carrots
½ cup minced fresh parsley
½ cup raisins
¼ cup blanched, sliced almonds
2 scallions, white and green parts
   thinly sliced
¼ cup diced red onion
1½ teaspoons Sesame Salt
   (page 254)

1. In a small nonstick skillet, melt the butter until sizzling, then add the curry powder. Stir for several minutes, being careful not to burn the butter. Place the couscous in a medium-size bowl. Pour enough of the boiling water into the pan with the sautéed curry powder to mix it with the water and rinse out the pan. Pour that and the remaining boiling water over the couscous. Cover tightly and allow the couscous to sit for 5 minutes. Fluff with a fork.
2. Mix together the yogurt, olive oil, vinegar, turmeric, lemon zest, and pepper; pour over the fluffed couscous, and mix well. Add the carrots, parsley, raisins, almonds, scallions, red onion, and sesame salt; mix well. Serve at room temperature.

❀ Curry It Up

There's a big difference in taste between "raw" curry powder and that which has been toasted or sautéed. Sautéing curry powder boosts the flavors, releasing the natural aromatic oils in the spices. One alternative is to use the Curry Powder from the recipe on page 263, which consists of spices that are toasted before they're ground.

Grilled Mushroom and Vegetable Medley

Spectrum Naturals Canola Spray
  Oil with Butter Flavor
1 large red bell pepper, seeded
1 large green bell pepper, seeded
2 medium-size zucchini
2 medium-size yellow squashes
2 cups fresh button mushrooms
4 medium-size green onions, white
  and green parts minced

1 teaspoon dried thyme
1 teaspoon dried basil
½ teaspoon garlic powder
¼ teaspoon mustard powder
⅛ teaspoon freshly ground black
  pepper
Optional: Vinaigrette dressing of
  choice

Serves 4	
Per serving:	
Calories:	31.27
Protein:	2.45 g
Carbohydrates:	6.44 g
Total fat:	0.31 g
Sat. fat:	0.06 g
Cholesterol:	0.00 mg
Sodium:	5.71 mg
Fiber:	2.19 g

1. Prepare a 20" × 14" sheet of heavy-duty foil by spraying the center with the spray oil.

2. Cut the bell peppers into ¼" strips; slice the zucchini and squashes cross-wise into ¼" slices. Slice the mushrooms. Arrange the vegetables over the foil. Evenly sprinkle the green onions, thyme, basil, garlic and mustard powders, and black pepper over the vegetables. Lightly spray the mixture with the spray oil. Fold the ends of the foil up and over the vegetables, wrapping it into a packet and sealing it by crimping the edges well, leaving space for heat to circulate.

3. Grill on a covered grill over medium coals for 20 to 25 minutes, or until the vegetables are fork tender. Carefully open the foil packet and grill for an additional 5 minutes to let the juices from the vegetables evaporate, if desired.

Stir-Fried Singapore Noodles

Serves 6	
Per serving:	
Calories:	265.75
Protein:	4.44 g
Carbohydrates:	39.09 g
Total fat:	10.43 g
Sat. fat:	1.66 g
Cholesterol:	35.47 mg
Sodium:	173.60 mg
Fiber:	2.69 g

¼ teaspoon freshly ground pepper
⅛ teaspoon Oriental mustard powder
¼ cup roasted red bell pepper, finely minced (see instructions for roasting red peppers on page 58)
1 teaspoon Bragg Liquid Aminos or low-sodium soy sauce
8 ounces vermicelli rice noodles
¼ cup sesame or vegetable oil, divided
1 tablespoon curry powder
1 teaspoon turmeric powder
¼ teaspoon Minor's Low Sodium Chicken Base
½ cup, plus 2 tablespoons water

1 small red or sweet onion, thinly sliced
3 cloves garlic, sliced
3 small shallots, sliced
½ cup broccoli florets
½ cup cauliflower florets
4 large carrots, peeled and shredded
1 cup thinly sliced napa cabbage
2 red chilies (or to taste), seeded and minced
1 large egg, beaten
Optional: 1 teaspoon honey
4 scallions, white and light green parts only, thinly sliced

1. Add the pepper, mustard powder, roasted red bell peppers, and Liquid Aminos to a small bowl; use a fork to mash together and mix well. Set aside. Place the rice noodles in enough lukewarm water to cover. Let soak until soft, about 20 minutes. Drain, and set aside.

2. Heat 2 tablespoons of the oil in a small nonstick sauté pan over medium heat. Add the curry and turmeric, and cook for 1 to 2 minutes or until fragrant. Add the chicken base; stir to dissolve in the oil. Add the roasted red pepper mixture and ½ cup of the water; mix well. Remove from heat and set aside.

3. In a wok or large, deep nonstick sauté pan, heat the remaining oil over medium-high heat. Add the onions, garlic, and shallots; stir-fry until just wilted, about 1 to 2 minutes, stirring constantly to prevent the garlic from burning. Add the broccoli and cauliflower, and stir-fry for 1 minute. Add the 2 tablespoons water; stir to combine. Add the carrots, napa cabbage, and chilies; cook until the vegetables are al dente, about 2 minutes.

4. Push the vegetables to the side to make a well in the bottom of the wok. Add the egg. Scramble until almost set, then incorporate into the other ingredients. Push the vegetables to the side again to make a well in the bottom of the wok and add the roasted red pepper mixture. Bring to temperature, then mix thoroughly to combine with the vegetables. Taste the vegetables at this point; if the taste is hotter than you prefer, add the honey to mellow the flavor. Add the drained, soaked noodles and toss to combine. Cook to heat through. Stir in the scallions. Transfer to serving platter. Serve immediately.

❈ Hot and Mellow

To turn Stir-Fried Singapore Noodles into a meatless main dish, you can substitute Mushroom Broth (page 164) or sake for the Minor's base and ½ cup of the water. Another way to turn this into a meatless dish and mellow the hotness of the chili is to use ½ cup apple juice as the liquid.

Oven-Roasted Corn on the Cob

Serves 4	
Per serving:	
Calories:	125.70
Protein:	4.69 g
Carbohydrates:	28.00 g
Total fat:	1.71 g
Sat. fat:	0.27 g
Cholesterol:	0.00 mg
Sodium:	21.73 mg
Fiber:	4.02 g

4 ears fresh sweet corn
4 teaspoons fresh lime juice

Freshly ground black pepper

1. Preheat oven to 350°.
2. Peel back the corn husks. Remove any silk. Brush the corn with the lime juice and generously grind black pepper over the corn. Pull the husks back up over the corn, twisting the husks at the top to keep them sealed.
3. Place the corn on the rack in a roasting pan large enough to hold the ears without overlapping. Roast for 30 minutes or until the corn is heated through and tender. Peel back the husks and use them as a handle, if desired, or discard the husks and insert corn holders into the ends of the cobs. Serve immediately.

❀ Slow-Simmer Flavor Without the (Time-Consuming) Fuss
You can enhance the flavor and add slow-simmered goodness to any recipe that includes tomato if you sauté the tomato (or tomato paste) for a few minutes until it takes on a caramel brown color. In a fraction of the time it usually takes to slow-simmer the sauce, sautéing the tomato adds a similar flavor dimension.

Oven-Fried Potato Wedges

*Spectrum Naturals Extra-Virgin
    Olive Spray Oil*
*4 large baking potatoes, washed
    and cut into 6 wedges each*
¾ teaspoon ground black pepper

1 teaspoon garlic powder
½ teaspoon dried rosemary, crushed
*½ teaspoon dried lemon granules,
    crushed*

Serves 4	
Per serving:	
Calories:	328.29
Protein:	6.88 g
Carbohydrates:	75.41 g
Total fat:	0.58 g
Sat. fat:	0.12 g
Cholesterol:	0.00 mg
Sodium:	23.91 mg
Fiber:	7.17 g

1. Preheat the oven to 400°.
2. Spray a baking sheet with the olive oil spray. Arrange the potato wedges on the sheet. Spray the potatoes with a thin layer of the olive oil spray. Sprinkle the potatoes with the pepper, garlic powder, rosemary, and lemon granules.
3. Bake for 30 to 35 minutes, turning the potatoes to the other cut side after 20 minutes. Bake until the potatoes are lightly browned, crisp outside, and tender inside.

Herb-Seasoned Roasted Red Onions

4 medium-size red onions
¼ teaspoon salt
4 teaspoons unsalted butter
⅛ teaspoon dried thyme

⅛ teaspoon dried parsley
⅛ teaspoon dried basil
⅛ teaspoon dried rosemary

Serves 4	
Per serving:	
Calories:	76.70
Protein:	1.35 g
Carbohydrates:	9.72 g
Total fat:	4.04 g
Sat. fat:	2.43 g
Cholesterol:	10.37 mg
Sodium:	149.36 mg
Fiber:	2.11 g

1. Preheat oven to 400°.
2. Remove the first layer of skin from the onions. Use a knife to cut off the bottom of the core end of each onion to give it a flat base. Make 2 cross-shaped cuts in the top of each onion, cutting halfway down. Stand the onions up in a ovenproof baking pan treated with nonstick spray. Sprinkle the onions with the salt, trying to get some into each "gap."
3. In a small bowl, mix the butter, thyme, parsley, basil, and rosemary. Divide the butter between the onions, placing it in the cross-cut slits of each onion. Bake for 30 to 35 minutes or until the onions are tender.

Golden Delicious Risotto

Serves 4	
Per serving:	
Calories:	334.99
Protein:	4.67 g
Carbohydrates:	49.43 g
Total fat:	13.66 g
Sat. fat:	5.09 g
Cholesterol:	17.75 mg
Sodium:	119.09 mg
Fiber:	1.45 g

4–5 cups water
2 tablespoons extra-virgin olive oil
2 tablespoons minced onion or
    shallot
1 cup arborio rice (short-grain
    white rice)
2 medium-size Golden Delicious
    apples, peeled, cored, and diced
¾ teaspoon Minor's Low Sodium
    Chicken Base

¼ teaspoon Minor's Sautéed
    Vegetable Base
⅓ cup dry white wine
2 tablespoons unsalted butter
2 tablespoons grated Parmesan
    cheese
Optional: Freshly grated nutmeg

1. In a medium-size saucepan, heat the water to boiling; reduce heat to maintain a steady simmer.
2. In a large nonstick sauté pan treated with nonstick spray, bring the olive oil to temperature over medium heat; add the onion (or shallot) and sauté for 3 minutes. Add the rice and half of the diced apple; sauté, stirring well, for 3 minutes. Add the bases and stir to dissolve. Add the wine and stir until the wine evaporates.
3. Stirring, ladle in enough of the water to just cover the rice (about ¾ cup). Lower the heat to maintain a steady simmer and cook the rice, stirring constantly, until almost all of the water has been absorbed, about 4 minutes.
4. Continue adding water ½ cup at a time, stirring, and cooking until absorbed. (The simmering water is added in small increments because you only want to use as much as is necessary for the rice to absorb before it's cooked; humidity and differences in burner temperature can make the difference in the amount of water needed.) After 15 minutes, stir in the remaining diced apples. The rice is done when it is creamy yet firm in the center (al dente). Total cooking time will be around 25 to 30 minutes.
5. Remove pan from heat; stir in the butter and Parmesan cheese. Serve immediately; grate nutmeg over the top of each serving, if desired.

Savory Vegetable Frittata

*1 cup zucchini, seeded and
   shredded*
*Spectrum Naturals Extra-Virgin
   Olive Spray Oil or other nonstick spray*
2 teaspoons olive oil
*2 teaspoons unsalted butter,
   melted and cooled*
1 stalk celery, finely minced
4 carrots, peeled and grated
1 large onion, sliced

4 large eggs
⅛ cup water
¼ teaspoon dried parsley
*⅛ teaspoon freshly ground black
   pepper*
Pinch chili powder
Pinch mustard powder
Pinch dried red pepper flakes
¼ cup grated Parmesan cheese
Optional: Freshly grated nutmeg

Serves 4	
Per serving:	
Calories:	178.73
Protein:	9.97 g
Carbohydrates:	9.88 g
Total fat:	11.22 g
Sat. fat:	4.27 g
Cholesterol:	222.62 mg
Sodium:	219.94 mg
Fiber:	2.33 g

1. Place the grated zucchini between several layers of paper towels and squeeze out the water; set aside.

2. Treat a large nonstick, ovenproof sauté pan with a thin coating of the spray oil. Bring to temperature over medium heat. Add the olive oil and butter. When the butter sizzles, add the celery and carrots; sauté for 3 minutes or until almost tender. Add the onion and zucchini; sauté, stirring occasionally, for 5 minutes or until the onion is transparent and moisture from the zucchini has evaporated from the pan.

3. Whisk together the eggs and water, then stir in the parsley, pepper, chili powder, mustard powder, and red pepper flakes. Pour the mixture over the sautéed vegetables in the pan. Tilt the pan so the eggs run around to the edges. Use a spoon or spatula to gently stir the eggs into the vegetables so that some of the eggs run to the bottom of the pan. Cook the eggs for about 3 minutes or until they begin to set in the center.

4. Remove from heat and sprinkle the Parmesan cheese evenly over the top of the frittata. Place the pan under the broiler for 1 to 2 minutes, until the cheese is melted and lightly browned. Watch carefully to avoid burning the frittata. Gently lift the edges of the frittata away from the pan with a spatula. Jiggle the pan to loosen the frittata, then slide it onto a serving platter. Use a knife or pizza cutter to cut the frittata into wedges. Serve with nutmeg freshly grated over the top, if desired.

Colcannon

Serves 4	
Per serving:	
Calories:	267.06
Protein:	7.05 g
Carbohydrates:	51.02 g
Total fat:	5.77 g
Sat. fat:	1.74 g
Cholesterol:	5.49 mg
Sodium:	436.87 mg
Fiber:	10.99 g

4 medium-size potatoes, peeled
   and cut into small dice
2 teaspoons lemon juice
2 teaspoons olive oil
1 small sweet onion, finely diced
1 tablespoon finely diced shallots
   or leeks
1 large green onion, white and
   green parts finely sliced
1 clove garlic, minced

1 small head green cabbage,
   cored and finely shredded
¼ teaspoon caraway seeds
2 teaspoons unsalted butter
¼ cup skim milk, scalded
¼ teaspoon dried parsley
⅛ teaspoon freshly ground black
   pepper
Optional: Fresh chives, chopped

1. Put the potatoes in a saucepan. Cover with cold water. Add the lemon juice and bring to a boil; reduce heat, cover, and simmer until tender.

2. In a large, deep nonstick sauté pan treated with nonstick spray, bring the olive oil to temperature over medium-high heat. Add the onion, shallots (or leeks), and green onion; sauté for about 3 minutes, stirring occasionally, until the onion is tender. Lower the heat and add the garlic; sauté for 1 minute. Add the cabbage and caraway seeds. Cover and cook until the cabbage is tender, about 10 minutes.

3. Drain the potatoes and put them in a serving dish large enough to hold all the ingredients. Add the butter, milk, parsley, and pepper; coarse-mash and mix with a fork. Add the sautéed cabbage mixture to the potatoes and stir to combine. Garnish with chives, if desired.

Roasted Butternut Squash

1 large butternut squash

Preheat oven to 350°. Wash the outside skin of the squash. Place the whole squash on a jelly roll pan or baking sheet. Pierce the skin a few times with a knife. Bake for 1 hour or until tender. Once the squash is cool enough to handle, slice it open, scrape out the seeds, and scrape the squash pulp off of the skin.

Serves 4	
Per ½-cup serving:	
Calories:	41.00
Protein:	0.92 g
Carbohydrates:	10.75 g
Total fat:	0.09 g
Sat. fat:	0.02 g
Cholesterol:	0.00 mg
Sodium:	4.10 mg
Fiber:	3.00 g

Sweet Potato Mash

4 medium-size sweet potatoes, peeled and cubed
2 teaspoons lemon juice
4 teaspoons unsalted butter
¼ teaspoon ground cumin
¼ teaspoon ground cinnamon
¼ teaspoon dried ginger
Optional: ¼ teaspoon chipotle powder or other salt-free chili powder
½ cup skim milk

1. Put the sweet potatoes in a saucepan. Cover with cold water. Add the lemon juice. Bring to a boil over medium heat. Cover and cook for 7 to 10 minutes, until the potatoes are fork tender. Once the sweet potatoes are fully cooked, drain the water from the pot and place them in a medium-size bowl.
2. Melt the butter in the saucepan over medium heat. Add the cumin, cinnamon, ginger, and chipotle powder; sauté the spices for 30 seconds. Add the milk and bring to a boil. Pour over the cooked sweet potatoes. Mix together using a masher or wooden spoon. Serve immediately.

Serves 4	
Per serving:	
Calories:	203.84
Protein:	3.59 g
Carbohydrates:	38.37 g
Total fat:	4.35 g
Sat. fat:	2.52 g
Cholesterol:	10.98 mg
Sodium:	36.10 mg
Fiber:	2.73 g

Roasted and Glazed Root Vegetables

Serves 4	
Per serving:	
Calories:	146.58
Protein:	2.91 g
Carbohydrates:	35.36 g
Total fat:	0.47 g
Sat. fat:	0.08 g
Cholesterol:	0.00 mg
Sodium:	98.29 mg
Fiber:	6.37 g

Spectrum Naturals Canola Spray Oil with Butter Flavor
4 small beets, peeled and diced
2 small white turnips, peeled and diced
4 large carrots, peeled and sliced
2 parsnips, peeled and diced
4 cloves garlic, minced
1 tablespoon candied ginger, snipped
4 teaspoons honey
¼ teaspoon (or to taste) freshly ground pepper
Garnish: chopped watercress

1. Preheat the oven to 350°.
2. Prepare the vegetables. Spray a jelly roll pan with the spray oil. Arrange the vegetables in a single layer across the pan. Sprinkle the garlic and ginger over the vegetables. Spray lightly with the spray oil.
3. Bake for 30 minutes. Drizzle the honey over the top of the vegetables. Use a spatula to stir the vegetables and then spread them back out into a single layer across the pan. Sprinkle with the ground pepper. Bake for an additional 15 minutes or until the vegetables are fork tender.
4. Transfer the vegetables to a serving bowl, stirring well to mix; toss with chopped watercress, if desired.

❀ Fat Primer
Like salt, fat is a nutrient you need; however, what is often misunderstood about fat is that it's the refined products like hydrogenated oils you should avoid. Some oils are chemically extracted—to avoid this, stick with cold-pressed oils for the healthiest choice.

East Meets West Corn

2 tablespoons ghee (clarified butter), divided

1 teaspoon yellow mustard seeds

1/8 teaspoon fenugreek seeds

1/4 teaspoon dried red pepper flakes

1/4 teaspoon ground ginger

1/2 teaspoon asafetida

1 large sweet onion, chopped

1 red bell pepper, seeded and chopped

1 green bell pepper, seeded and chopped

2 cloves garlic, minced

1/4 teaspoon turmeric

2 jalapeño peppers, seeded and chopped

2 (10-ounce) packages Cascadian Farm frozen Organic Super Sweet Corn, thawed

2 tablespoons freeze-dried shallot

1 teaspoon freeze-dried cilantro

2½ cups plain nonfat yogurt

Serves 8	
Per serving:	
Calories:	147.64
Protein:	7.17 g
Carbohydrates:	24.09 g
Total fat:	4.26 g
Sat. fat:	2.35 g
Cholesterol:	11.41 mg
Sodium:	55.58 mg
Fiber:	2.30 g

1. Bring a large, deep nonstick sauté pan to temperature over medium heat. Melt 1 teaspoon of the ghee. Add the mustard and fenugreek seeds. Cover (because the mustard seeds will pop) and toast for 30 seconds, jiggling the pan to move the spices and prevent them from scorching. Transfer to a mortar and pestle along with the red pepper flakes and ginger; pound into a paste. Set aside.

2. Add the remaining ghee to the sauté pan. Add the asafetida and sauté for 1 minute over medium heat. Add the onion and bell peppers; sauté until the onion is transparent. Add the garlic and cook for 1 minute, stirring the garlic into the onion-pepper mixture. Add the turmeric and mustard-seed paste; stir into the onion mixture. (Add 1 or 2 tablespoons of water at this point if the mixture is dry.)

3. Add the jalapeño peppers and corn; stir-fry with the onion-pepper mixture, cooking for 2 minutes. Stir in the shallot, cilantro, and yogurt. Lower the heat and simmer, covered, for 5 minutes. Serve immediately.

Butternut Squash Cheese Muffins

Serves 12	
Per serving:	
Calories:	88.02
Protein:	3.59 g
Carbohydrates:	8.84 g
Total fat:	4.83 g
Saturated Fat:	1.76 g
Cholesterol:	42.17 mg
Sodium:	85.33 mg
Fiber:	0.79 g

1 tablespoon unsalted butter

1 tablespoon extra-light olive oil or canola oil

1 cup chopped sweet onion

1 cup sliced button mushrooms

¼ cup water

2 cups cubed Roasted Butternut Squash (page 181)

6 tablespoons unbleached all-purpose flour

3 tablespoons oat bran or wheat germ

2 large eggs

¼ teaspoon freshly ground black pepper

½ cup grated Jarlsberg cheese

1 tablespoon hulled sesame seeds

1. Preheat oven to 400°.
2. Add the butter and oil to a nonstick sauté pan over high heat. When the butter begins to sizzle, reduce heat to medium and add the onion and mushrooms. Sauté until the onion is transparent. Set aside to cool.
3. In the bowl of a food processor or in a blender, combine the cooled sautéed mixture and all of the remaining ingredients *except* the cheese and sesame seeds; pulse until mixed.
4. Fold the cheese into the squash mixture. Spoon the resulting batter into muffin cups treated with nonstick spray (or lined with foil muffin liners), filling each muffin section to the top. Evenly divide the sesame seeds over the top of the batter. Bake for 35 to 40 minutes. (For savory appetizers, make 24 minimuffins; bake for 20 to 25 minutes.)

French-Glazed Green Beans

Serves 4	
Per serving:	
Calories:	127.39
Protein:	2.91 g
Carbohydrates:	10.26 g
Total fat:	9.61 g
Sat. fat:	0.92 g
Cholesterol:	0.00 mg
Sodium:	30.96 mg
Fiber:	3.80 g

¼ cup chopped walnuts

4 teaspoons cold-pressed walnut or canola oil

2 (15-ounce) cans French-cut green beans

1 teaspoon lemon juice

1 teaspoon honey

1 teaspoon French Spice Blend (page 276)

⅛ teaspoon dried lemon granules, crushed

⅛ teaspoon mustard powder

⅛ teaspoon freshly ground black pepper

1. Bring a large, deep nonstick sauté pan to temperature over medium heat. Add the walnuts. Toast for 3 minutes, stirring frequently so the walnuts don't burn. Transfer to a bowl and set aside.

2. Add the walnut oil to the pan. Drain the green beans and add to the pan; stir to toss in the oil. Once the green beans are brought to temperature, push them to the sides of the pan. Add the lemon juice, honey, spice blend, lemon granules, mustard powder, and pepper; stir to combine. Toss the green beans in the lemon juice mixture. Pour into a serving bowl and top with the toasted walnuts.

❀ Go Organic!

There are other advantages to organic cooking and salad oils in addition to the absence of pesticide and chemical fertilizers used during the growing process (and thus no residue from them in the products) and the absence of preservatives added to the products later: Many commercial oils are extracted using hexane or other chemicals. Organic cold-pressed and expeller-pressed vegetable oils are easier for the body to digest, so they're the healthier choices.

Vegetables in Warm Citrus Vinaigrette

Serves 4	
Per serving:	
Calories:	48.27
Protein:	1.73 g
Carbohydrates:	5.99 g
Total fat:	2.25 g
Sat. fat:	0.22 g
Cholesterol:	0.00 mg
Sodium:	21.19 mg
Fiber:	1.67 g

Pinch saffron
Pinch lemon or lime zest (or dried lemon or lime granules, crushed)
2 teaspoons Spectrum Naturals Grapeseed Oil
1 tablespoon water
Spectrum Naturals Grapeseed Spray Oil
1 (10-ounce) package Cascadian Farm frozen Organic California Blend Vegetables, thawed
1 tablespoon Cascadian Farm Frozen Organic Orange Juice Concentrate
⅛ teaspoon freshly ground black pepper

1. Preheat oven to 350°.
2. Add the saffron, zest, grapeseed oil, and water to a microwave-safe bowl. Microwave on high for 20 to 30 seconds, until the water just boils; stir. Cover and set aside to infuse at room temperature while the vegetables bake.
3. Treat an ovenproof casserole dish with the spray oil. Add the thawed vegetables. Spray a light coating of additional spray oil over the top of the vegetables. Cover and bake for 15 minutes. Carefully remove the cover and stir the vegetables. Spray with an additional coating of the spray oil. Bake for an additional 15 minutes.
4. During the last few minutes of the baking time, add the frozen orange juice concentrate to the saffron-oil mixture. Whisk to combine.
5. Remove the vegetables from the oven. Pour the saffron-orange vinaigrette over the vegetables and add the pepper; toss to combine. Serve immediately.

❊ Concentrate on Your Cooking

You can substitute reduced fresh orange juice for the frozen fruit juice concentrate and water called for in the Vegetables in Warm Citrus Vinaigrette. Using a frozen fruit juice concentrate saves some time, however, because you can simply mix it for the strength you need.

Curried Sweet Potato Latkes

Spectrum Naturals Canola Spray
   Oil with Butter Flavor
2 teaspoons ghee
1/4 teaspoon cayenne
1/4 teaspoon ground cinnamon
2 teaspoons curry powder
1 teaspoon ground cumin
1 3/4 pounds sweet potatoes or
   yams, peeled and grated
1 medium-size sweet onion, finely
   chopped
1/4 teaspoon salt

1/4 teaspoon dried lemon granules,
   crushed
1/4 teaspoon freshly ground white
   or black pepper
1 teaspoon low-salt baking powder
2 teaspoons granulated sugar
1 teaspoon brown sugar
2 large eggs plus 1 large egg
   white, lightly beaten together
1/3 cup unbleached all-purpose flour
1 teaspoon canola oil

Serves 4	
Per serving:	
Calories:	156.26
Protein:	4.08 g
Carbohydrates:	27.81 g
Total fat:	3.31 g
Sat. fat:	1.24 g
Cholesterol:	56.46 mg
Sodium:	173.62 mg
Fiber:	1.85 g

1. Preheat oven to 350°. Treat a baking sheet with the canola oil spray.
2. Bring a small nonstick sauté pan to temperature over medium-high heat. Melt the ghee in the skillet, then add the cayenne, cinnamon, curry powder, and cumin. Sauté the spices, stirring constantly, for 30 seconds. Remove from heat.
3. In a large bowl, mix together the sautéed spice mixture and all the remaining ingredients. Spoon the batter onto the prepared baking sheet in 8 equal-sized portions, flattening them slightly. Spray the tops of the pancakes with a light coating of the spray oil.
4. Bake for 15 minutes or until brown on the bottom. Turn and bake for an additional 10 to 15 minutes, until evenly browned. Serve immediately.

Cauliflower in Ginger Cheese Sauce

Serves 4	
Per serving:	
Calories:	191.68
Protein:	10.95 g
Carbohydrates:	7.72 g
Total fat:	13.60 g
Sat. fat:	6.97 g
Cholesterol:	33.90 mg
Sodium:	348.11 mg
Fiber:	2.22 g

2 cups cauliflower, cooked
2 teaspoons unsalted butter
2 teaspoons canola oil
1 clove garlic, minced
¾ teaspoon ground ginger
2 teaspoons unbleached all-purpose flour
½ cup skim milk

1 tablespoon instant nonfat dry milk
¼ teaspoon Dijon mustard
1 tablespoon freeze-dried shallots
½ cup grated sharp Cheddar cheese
½ cup grated Swiss cheese

1. Prepare the cauliflower and keep warm.
2. Bring a small nonstick saucepan to temperature over medium heat. Add the oil and butter. Once the butter begins to sizzle, add the garlic and ginger; sauté for 1 minute, stirring to mix the garlic with the ginger and to prevent the garlic from burning. Add the flour and stir to blend with the oil and butter.
3. Whisk together the milk, dry milk, and mustard. Slowly add the milk mixture to the pan, stirring constantly to mix it into the flour-butter roux. Increase the heat to medium-high and bring the milk to a boil, stirring constantly. Immediately lower the heat to medium-low. Simmer the mixture while continuing to stir, and add the shallots.
4. Once the mixture thickens, remove the pan from the burner. Add the cheese. Stir constantly until the cheese is melted. Pour over the cooked cauliflower and serve immediately.

❀ Cheese Sauce Primer

When making the Cauliflower in Ginger Cheese Sauce recipe, it's important that the thickened milk isn't too warm once you get ready to add the cheese; too hot of a temperature will cause the oils in the cheese to separate. Also, the skim milk and nonfat dry milk mixture will scorch more easily than will whole milk or cream.

Baked Stuffed Tomatoes

1¼ cups chopped parsley
3 small cloves garlic, finely
  chopped
Pinch red pepper flakes
¾ cup bread crumbs
Spectrum Naturals Extra-Virgin
  Olive Spray Oil

10 plum tomatoes, cut in half
  lengthwise and seeded
½ teaspoon freshly ground black
  pepper
¼ teaspoon dried lemon granules,
  crushed
½ cup water

Serves 4	
Per serving:	
Calories:	118.79
Protein:	4.81 g
Carbohydrates:	24.38 g
Total fat:	1.91 g
Sat. fat:	0.27 g
Cholesterol:	0.08 mg
Sodium:	93.43 mg
Fiber:	4.06 g

1. Preheat oven to 400°.
2. In the bowl of a food processor, combine the parsley, garlic, red pepper flakes, and bread crumbs; pulse to chop and mix. Set aside.
3. Prepare a casserole dish or baking pan large enough to hold the tomato halves side by side by spraying it with the olive oil spray. Fill the tomato halves with the bread crumb mixture and place them in the dish or pan. Spray a light layer of the olive spray oil over the tops of the filled tomatoes. Sprinkle the pepper and lemon granules over the top of the bread crumbs.
4. Add ½ cup water to the bottom of the pan. Cover tightly with an aluminum foil tent. Bake for 45 minutes or until the tomatoes are tender.
5. Remove the aluminum foil. Place the pan under the broiler and broil until crisp and slightly browned, about 2 minutes. (Watch closely so the bread crumbs don't burn!)

❈ Using Less Fat

When you use cold-pressed vegetable oil in a recipe that calls for butter, you can usually reduce the amount of oil you use by 25 percent. In other words, if the recipe calls for 1 teaspoon of butter, you'll only need to use ¾ teaspoon of oil.

Caribbean Corn on the Cob

Serves 4	
Per serving:	
Calories:	79.48
Protein:	2.93 g
Carbohydrates:	17.81 g
Total fat:	1.07 g
Sat. fat:	0.16 g
Cholesterol:	0.00 mg
Sodium:	13.58 mg
Fiber:	2.46 g

4 cups water
⅛ cup lime juice
1 teaspoon Caribbean Spice Blend (page 275)

4 medium-size ears yellow sweet corn
Optional: Freshly ground black pepper

In a large, deep nonstick sauté pan, bring the water to a boil. Stir in the lime juice and the seasoning. Add the corn. Cover, reduce heat, and simmer for 8 minutes, turning the corn occasionally. Serve topped with freshly ground black pepper, if desired.

Carrots with an English Accent

Serves 4	
Per serving:	
Calories:	70.52
Protein:	1.70 g
Carbohydrates:	16.46 g
Total fat:	0.28 g
Sat. fat:	0.05 g
Cholesterol:	0.00 mg
Sodium:	102.97 mg
Fiber:	5.15 g

Spectrum Naturals Canola Spray Oil with Butter Flavor
¼ cup water
1 teaspoon lemon juice

4 cups baby carrots, sliced
1 teaspoon English Spice Blend (page 276)

1. Preheat oven to 350°.
2. Treat an ovenproof casserole dish with the spray oil. Add the water and lemon juice, and stir to combine. Spread the carrot slices over the water-lemon mixture. Mist the carrots with the spray oil. Sprinkle the seasoning over the carrots. Cover and bake for 45 minutes. Mist the carrots again with the spray oil, if desired. Uncover and bake for an additional 10 minutes or until the carrots are tender.

Curried Parsnip Purée

6 parsnips, peeled and cut into
  ½" cubes
1 teaspoon Hot Curry Spice Blend
  (page 277)

4 teaspoons unsalted butter
½ cup warm skim milk

1. Cook the parsnip cubes in gently boiling water for 12 minutes or until tender. Drain well.
2. Add the parsnips to the bowl of a food processor along with the remaining ingredients; process until smooth.

Serves 4	
Per serving:	
Calories:	228.34
Protein:	3.21 g
Carbohydrates:	46.88 g
Total fat:	4.56 g
Sat. fat:	2.51 g
Cholesterol:	10.37 mg
Sodium:	24.52 mg
Fiber:	9.60 g

Middle Eastern Glazed Carrots

4 cups sliced carrots
2 teaspoons canola oil
2 teaspoons unsalted butter
1 teaspoon Middle Eastern Spice
  Blend (page 274)

2 teaspoons granulated sugar
⅛ teaspoon freshly ground black
  pepper

1. Put the carrots in a microwave-safe casserole dish. Cover and microwave on high for 3 minutes; turn the dish. Microwave on high for 4 minutes or until the carrots are tender.
2. Bring a large, deep nonstick sauté pan to temperature over medium heat. Add the oil, butter, and spice blend; sauté the spices for 1 minute. Add the carrots and stir to mix. Sprinkle the sugar and pepper over the carrots and stir-fry until the carrots are heated through and the sugar forms a glaze.

Serves 4	
Per serving:	
Calories:	115.19
Protein:	1.72 g
Carbohydrates:	18.45 g
Total fat:	4.45 g
Sat. fat:	1.41 g
Cholesterol:	5.18 mg
Sodium:	103.24 mg
Fiber:	5.15 g

Quinoa and Artichoke Pilaf

Serves 4	
Per serving:	
Calories:	248.90
Protein:	8.56 g
Carbohydrates:	46.57 g
Total fat:	4.81 g
Sat. fat:	0.61 g
Cholesterol:	0.05 mg
Sodium:	235.74 mg
Fiber:	7.13 g

2 cups water
1 teaspoon Minor's Roasted
   Mirepoix Flavor Concentrate
1 cup quinoa, rinsed
1 bay leaf
½ teaspoon turmeric
¼ teaspoon pepper
1 tablespoon olive oil
⅛ teaspoon dried lemon granules,
   crushed

1 large tomato, peeled and finely
   chopped
1 (9-ounce) package frozen no-salt-
   added artichoke hearts, thawed
   and quartered
1 small red onion, diced
½ cup canned pitted black olives,
   rinsed and drained
¼ cup currants

1. In a large, deep nonstick sauté pan over medium heat, combine the water, flavor concentrate, quinoa, bay leaf, turmeric, pepper, olive oil, and lemon granules. Cover and simmer for 15 to 20 minutes, until the water is absorbed.
2. Remove from heat. Remove and discard the bay leaf, then add the tomato, artichokes, onion, olives, and currants; stir to combine. Serve immediately.

❀ Quinoa Primer
Quinoa is a South American high-protein grain that is considered a complete protein because it contains all 8 essential amino acids. The tiny round "granules" make an excellent reduced-carb rice substitute. It cooks in about half the time of rice.

Baked Cajun Cauliflower

1¾-pound head cauliflower
1 teaspoon lemon juice
⅛ teaspoon mustard powder
Spectrum Naturals Canola Spray
    Oil with Butter Flavor

½–1 teaspoon Cajun Spice Blend
    (see page 274)

Serves 6	
Per serving:	
Calories:	30.64
Protein:	2.44 g
Carbohydrates:	5.51 g
Total fat:	0.60 g
Sat. fat:	0.09 g
Cholesterol:	0.00 mg
Sodium:	19.85 mg
Fiber:	3.58 g

1. Preheat oven to 375°.
2. Trim off the outer leaves of the cauliflower. Cut the base so that the head will sit upright. Bring a large pot of water to boil over medium-high heat. Add the lemon juice and mustard powder; stir to mix. Add the cauliflower, base down, and blanch for 5 minutes. Remove and drain.
3. Treat a deep ovenproof casserole dish with the spray oil. Place the cauliflower base down in the casserole dish. Lightly mist the cauliflower with the spray oil. Evenly sprinkle the Cajun Blend over the top of the cauliflower. Cover and bake for 15 minutes.

❈ Cajun Creativity

A touch of sweet applesauce can mellow the spiciness of Cajun seasoning. To create a savory-sweet vegetable entrée, mix the desired amount of Cajun Blend seasoning mixture with ⅛ cup unsweetened, no-salt-added applesauce to make a paste. Spread the paste over the cauliflower and bake according to the Baked Cajun Cauliflower directions.

Oven-Dried Seasoned Tomatoes

Serves 8	
Per serving:	
Calories:	6.51
Protein:	0.26 g
Carbohydrates:	1.44 g
Total fat:	0.10 g
Sat. fat:	0.01 g
Cholesterol:	0.00 mg
Sodium:	2.79 mg
Fiber:	0.34 g

4 plum tomatoes, peeled, seeded, and cut into quarters
Spectrum Naturals Extra-Virgin Olive Spray Oil
⅛ teaspoon freshly ground black pepper
½ teaspoon Pasta Blend (page 275)

1. Preheat oven to 250°.
2. Put the tomatoes in a bowl. Lightly mist with the spray oil, toss, and then mist again. Add the pepper and Pasta Blend. Arrange the tomatoes on a baking sheet and bake until somewhat dried, about 2½ to 3 hours.

Savory Stir-Fried Spinach

Serves 4	
Per serving:	
Calories:	109.73
Protein:	7.19 g
Carbohydrates:	11.85 g
Total fat:	5.36 g
Sat. fat:	0.46 g
Cholesterol:	0.00 mg
Sodium:	235.51 mg
Fiber:	6.60 g

4 teaspoons canola oil
1 large sweet onion, chopped
1 clove garlic
½ teaspoon Garam Masala Spice Blend (page 277)
2 pounds fresh spinach, washed and stems removed
1 tablespoon dry white wine
2 teaspoons Bragg Liquid Aminos
1 teaspoon minced candied ginger

1. Bring a large, deep nonstick sauté pan to temperature over medium heat. Add the oil and onion; sauté for 5 minutes or until the onion is transparent.
2. Add the garlic and Garam Masala Blend; stir to combine. Add the spinach and stir-fry for 3 minutes.
3. Add the wine, Liquid Aminos, and candied ginger; cover, reduce heat, and allow to steam for 4 minutes. Serve immediately.

Baked Potato Latkes

Spectrum Naturals Canola Spray
  Oil with Butter Flavor
4 medium-size potatoes, peeled and
  grated
1 medium-size red onion, finely
  chopped
¼ teaspoon salt
⅛ teaspoon dried lemon granules,
  crushed

½ teaspoon grated black pepper
1 teaspoon freeze-dried chives
1 large egg plus 1 large egg
  white, lightly beaten together
¼ cup unbleached all-purpose flour
1 teaspoon canola oil

Serves 8	
Per serving:	
Calories:	107.94
Protein:	3.30 g
Carbohydrates:	21.03 g
Total fat:	1.33 g
Sat. fat:	0.26 g
Cholesterol:	26.56 mg
Sodium:	141.26 mg
Fiber:	1.44 g

1. Preheat oven to 350°. Treat a baking sheet with the canola oil spray.
2. Mix together the remaining ingredients. Spoon the batter onto the baking sheet in 8 equal-sized portions, flattening them slightly. Spray the tops of the pancakes with a light coating of the canola spray oil.
3. Bake for 10 minutes or until brown on the bottom. Turn and bake for an additional 5 to 10 minutes, until evenly browned.

❀ Latke Cooking Tips

Always press as much water as possible out of the potatoes. One way to do this is to wrap the grated potatoes in several layers of paper towels and squeeze out the water. Lighter-tasting oils, like the recommended canola oil or grapeseed oil, are essential; otherwise, the flavors of the latkes can be overpowered by the taste of the oil. These recipes recommend the butter-flavored nonstick spray to add another layer of flavor to compensate for the small amount of salt used. If you prefer a more traditional-tasting latke, substitute unflavored canola or grapeseed oil spray for the butter-flavored spray.

Savory Zucchini Pancakes

Serves 4	
Per serving:	
Calories:	141.74
Protein:	9.07 g
Carbohydrates:	2.03 g
Total fat:	10.74 g
Sat. fat:	5.13 g
Cholesterol:	227.80 mg
Sodium:	180.80 mg
Fiber:	0.42 g

2 cups shredded zucchini, seeded
4 large eggs
4 teaspoons unsalted butter,
  melted and cooled
¼ cup grated Parmesan cheese
⅛ teaspoon ground black pepper

Pinch mustard powder
Spectrum Naturals Canola Spray
  Oil with Butter Flavor
Optional: Freshly grated nutmeg

1. Place the shredded zucchini between several layers of paper towels and squeeze out the water. Whisk the eggs, then stir in the butter, cheese, pepper, and mustard powder. Add the zucchini and mix well. Consistency should be that of a thick pancake batter. Adjust consistency with water, added 1 teaspoon at a time, if the batter is too thick.
2. Treat a large nonstick sauté pan or griddle with a thin coating of the spray oil. Bring to temperature over medium heat. Spoon the batter onto the pan and flatten with the back of a spoon. When lightly browned, flip. Continue until all the batter is used. (Pancakes can be placed on a baking sheet set in a warm oven to be kept warm.) Serve with freshly grated nutmeg over the top of the pancakes, if desired.

❋ Freezing Roasted Butternut Squash

In the fall, try to get several scrumptious butternut squashes from a local organic farmer. It's easy to make extra because up to 4 of them will fit on a jelly roll pan. Freeze any leftovers in fork-mashed, ½-cup increments, so they're ready to add to your favorite recipes or to season and heat for a vegetable side dish.

CHAPTER 11
Pasta and Pizza

Simple Tomato Sauce

½ cup extra-virgin olive oil
1 large sweet onion, chopped
2 cloves garlic, minced
1 large stalk celery, finely chopped
1 large carrot, peeled and grated
¼ teaspoon freshly ground black pepper
⅛ teaspoon mustard powder
1 (14.5-ounce) can Muir Glen Organic No Salt Added Diced Tomatoes
¼ teaspoon (or to taste) granulated sugar
⅛ teaspoon dried lemon granules, crushed
1 (15-ounce) can Muir Glen Organic No Salt Added Tomato Sauce
1 (28-ounce) can Muir Glen Organic No Salt Added Tomato Purée
2 dried bay leaves
½ teaspoon dried oregano, crushed
½ teaspoon dried basil, crushed
Pinch red pepper flakes
Optional: 1 teaspoon onion powder
Optional: 1 teaspoon garlic powder
Optional: 4 tablespoons unsalted butter or fine extra-virgin olive oil

1. In a large, deep nonstick sauté pan, heat the oil over medium-high heat. Add the onion and garlic; sauté until soft and translucent, about 5 to 10 minutes. Add the celery, carrots, black pepper, and mustard powder; mix well. Sauté for 5 minutes. Drain the juice from the diced tomatoes and reserve. Add the drained tomatoes to the pot; sauté until all the vegetables are soft, about 5 to 10 minutes. Add the sautéed tomato mixture to the bowl of a food processor; process until smooth. Return to the pan.

2. Add the reserved juice from the tomatoes, the sugar, lemon granules, tomato sauce, tomato purée, bay leaves, oregano, basil, and red pepper flakes; reduce heat and simmer, uncovered, for 45 minutes. Remove the bay leaves and check for seasoning, adding the garlic and onion powders at this time, if desired. Simmer for an additional 15 minutes or until thick. If the sauce tastes too acidic, add a little bit more sugar or some fresh or dried thyme, a pinch at a time; if you're not watching your fat and cholesterol, you can also mellow the flavor by whisking in some unsalted butter, 1 tablespoon at a time; otherwise, use fine extra-virgin olive oil.

Low-Fat Tomato Sauce

Spectrum Naturals Extra-Virgin
Olive Spray Oil
1 large sweet onion, chopped
2 cloves garlic, minced
1 large stalk celery, finely chopped
1 large carrot, peeled and grated
1 dried bay leaf
1 (14.5-ounce) can Muir Glen Organic
No Salt Added Diced Tomatoes
½ teaspoon dried oregano, crushed
½ teaspoon dried basil, crushed
Pinch red pepper flakes
¼ teaspoon ground black pepper

⅛ teaspoon mustard powder
1 teaspoon (or to taste) granulated sugar
⅛ teaspoon dried lemon granules,
crushed
1 (15-ounce) can Muir Glen Organic
No Salt Added Tomato Sauce
1 (28-ounce) can Muir Glen
Organic No Salt Added Tomato
Purée
1 teaspoon onion powder
1 teaspoon garlic powder
2 teaspoons extra-virgin olive oil

Serves 12	
Per serving:	
Calories:	56.19
Protein:	1.89 g
Carbohydrates:	11.89 g
Total fat:	0.79 g
Sat. fat:	0.11 g
Cholesterol:	0.00 mg
Sodium:	57.73 mg
Fiber:	2.33 g

1. In a large, covered microwave-safe casserole dish treated with the olive spray oil, add the onion, garlic, celery, carrots, and bay leaf. Drain the juice from the diced tomatoes and reserve. Add the drained tomatoes to the dish; mix well. Cover and microwave on high for 5 minutes, turning the dish halfway through the cooking time. Carefully remove the cover and stir in the oregano, basil, red pepper flakes, black pepper, mustard powder, sugar, and lemon granules. Cover and let rest for 3 minutes. Carefully remove the cover and check that the onion is transparent. If not, microwave on high for additional 1-minute increments until all the vegetables are cooked and soft.
2. Remove the bay leaf and add the sautéed tomato mixture to the bowl of a food processor; process until smooth.
3. Bring a large, deep nonstick sauté pan treated with the spray oil to temperature over low heat. Add the puréed tomato-vegetable mixture, reserved juice from the tomatoes, tomato sauce, and tomato purée; reduce heat and simmer, uncovered, for 45 minutes.
4. Add the garlic and onion powders; simmer for an additional 15 minutes or until thick. Whisk in the extra-virgin olive oil. If the sauce tastes too acidic, add a little bit more sugar or thyme, a pinch at a time.

Toasted Walnut and Parsley Pesto with Noodles

Serves 4	
Per serving:	
Calories:	398.31
Protein:	10.09 g
Carbohydrates:	42.05 g
Total fat:	21.62 g
Sat. fat:	2.64 g
Cholesterol:	54.60 mg
Sodium:	60.29 mg
Fiber:	2.66 g

4 tablespoons chopped walnuts

4 cups cooked egg noodles (no salt added to cooking water)

4 tablespoons Roland Walnut Oil or Extra-Virgin Olive Oil

¾ cup fresh parsley

2 tablespoons grated Parmesan cheese

1 clove garlic, crushed

2 teaspoons fresh lemon juice

Freshly ground black pepper, to taste

1. In a small nonstick saucepan over medium heat, toast the walnuts until they're light brown, being careful not to burn them. Set aside to cool.
2. Cook the noodles in unsalted water according to package directions. Drain.
3. While the noodles cook, add the oil, parsley, Parmesan cheese, crushed garlic, lemon juice, and half of the toasted walnuts to the bowl of a food processor. Process until smooth.
4. In a large serving bowl, toss the warm, drained cooked noodles with the pesto and the remaining chopped toasted walnuts. Grind the black pepper over the pasta and serve.

❀ Seasoning Suggestions

Even though some Mrs. Dash Classic Italiano or Tomato Basil Garlic Seasoning Blend is good sprinkled over the top of a serving of Toasted Walnut and Parsley Pesto with Noodles, be adventurous and try something out of the ordinary, like a Chipotle Chili Powder Spice Blend (page 277) or salt-free chili powder blend.

Spinach Ravioli in Tomato Mushroom Sauce

1 (10-ounce) package frozen no-salt-added chopped spinach, thawed and squeezed dry
¼ cup part-skim ricotta cheese
⅛ teaspoon freshly grated nutmeg
8 teaspoons Parmesan cheese, divided
8 egg roll wrappers (6½" squares)
2 large eggs, beaten with 1 teaspoon water

4 teaspoons extra-virgin olive oil, divided
2 cups fresh button mushrooms, sliced
2 cups Low-Fat Tomato Sauce (page 199)
Freshly ground black pepper
4 quarts water
1 tablespoon lemon juice

Serves 4	
Per serving:	
Calories:	387.39
Protein:	17.52 g
Carbohydrates:	56.29 g
Total fat:	11.31 g
Sat. fat:	3.11 g
Cholesterol:	119.45 mg
Sodium:	598.49 mg
Fiber:	6.48 g

1. Add the spinach, ricotta, nutmeg, and 4 teaspoons of the Parmesan cheese to a small bowl and mix well.
2. To fill the wonton wrappers and make the "ravioli," line half of the wrappers up on a cutting board. Brush with the egg and water mixture. Using a teaspoon, arrange a dollop of the filling on each wrapper. Place another wrapper directly on top, pressing around the filling and sealing the edges. Crimp the edges with a fork to make sure they're sealed completely. Place the ravioli onto a floured baking sheet and keep covered with a damp cotton towel.
3. Bring a large, deep nonstick sauté pan to temperature over medium heat. Add 3 teaspoons of the olive oil. Add the mushrooms; sauté for 3 to 5 minutes. Stir in the tomato sauce, black pepper to taste, and any remaining egg-water mixture; reduce heat and keep warm.
4. In a large pot, bring 4 quarts of water to a boil; add the lemon juice and the remaining 1 teaspoon oil. Carefully add small batches of ravioli, about 3 to 4 at a time. This will prevent them from crowding in the pot and sticking together. Cook for 2 to 3 minutes. Using a spider strainer or slotted spoon, carefully remove the ravioli and place on a plate. Tent with foil to keep warm while cooking the remaining ravioli.
5. Divide the cooked ravioli between 4 serving plates. Top with mushroom tomato sauce and sprinkle each serving with 1 teaspoon of the remaining freshly grated Parmesan cheese. Serve immediately.

Whole-Wheat Pasta in Bleu Cheese Sauce

Serves 4	
Per serving:	
Calories:	309.56
Protein:	16.32 g
Carbohydrates:	38.55 g
Total fat:	11.29 g
Sat. fat:	4.64 g
Cholesterol:	16.84 mg
Sodium:	320.93 mg
Fiber:	6.33 g

4 teaspoons olive oil
2 cloves garlic, minced
½ cup nonfat cottage cheese
2 ounces crumbled bleu cheese
Optional: Skim milk, as needed
4 cups cooked whole-wheat pasta
¼ cup freshly grated Parmesan cheese
Freshly ground black pepper
Optional: Dry-toasted chopped walnuts

1. Heat the olive oil in a large nonstick skillet. Add the garlic and sauté for 1 minute. Lower the heat, stir in the cottage cheese, and bring it to temperature. Add the bleu cheese and stir to combine; thin the sauce with a little skim milk, if necessary.
2. Toss with the pasta and divide into 4 equal servings. Top each serving with 1 tablespoon of the Parmesan cheese, freshly ground black pepper to taste, and toasted walnuts.

Garlic Toast with a Kick

Serves 4	
Per serving:	
Calories:	77.06
Protein:	2.31 g
Carbohydrates:	16.06 g
Total fat:	0.22 g
Sat. fat:	0.03 g
Cholesterol:	0.00 mg
Sodium:	24.85 mg
Fiber:	0.65 g

Spectrum Naturals Extra-Virgin Olive Spray Oil
8 (½-ounce) slices French Bread (page 216)
2 teaspoons garlic powder
½ teaspoon onion powder
¼ teaspoon ground ginger
¼ teaspoon sweet paprika
⅛ teaspoon dried parsley, crushed
⅛ teaspoon oregano, crushed
⅛ teaspoon mustard powder
⅛ teaspoon cumin
1/16 teaspoon dried red pepper flakes, crushed
1/16 teaspoon cayenne

Preheat oven to 350°. Using the spray oil, lightly spray both sides of each slice of bread. Arrange the bread slices on a baking sheet. Combine all the remaining ingredients; mix well. Sprinkle the spice mixture over the tops of the bread slices; press the seasoning into the bread and then lightly spray with the spray oil again. Bake for 6 to 8 minutes.

Spinach Pasta in Tuna Alfredo Sauce

1 cup nonfat cottage cheese
1 tablespoon skim milk
⅛ teaspoon freshly ground black
   pepper
⅛ teaspoon mustard powder
2 teaspoons olive oil
1 clove minced garlic

2 (6-ounce) cans Chicken of the
   Sea Very Low Sodium Tuna,
   drained
⅛ cup dry white wine
¼ cup freshly grated Parmesan
   cheese
4 cups cooked spinach pasta

Serves 4	
Per serving:	
Calories:	297.96
Protein:	25.78 g
Carbohydrates:	37.57 g
Total fat:	4.04 g
Sat. fat:	1.52 g
Cholesterol:	26.23 mg
Sodium:	167.31 mg
Fiber:	0.00 g

1. Add the cottage cheese, skim milk, pepper, and mustard powder to a food processor or blender container; process until smooth. Set aside.
2. Bring the olive oil to temperature in a large, deep nonstick sauté pan over medium heat. Add the garlic and sauté for 1 minute; stir in the tuna and sauté for 1 more minute. Add the wine to the skillet and bring to a boil.
3. Lower the heat and add the creamed cottage cheese; bring to temperature, being careful not to boil the sauce. Stir in the Parmesan cheese and continue to heat the sauce for another minute, stirring constantly. Add the pasta and toss with the sauce. Divide into 4 equal servings and serve immediately, topped with additional freshly ground pepper, if desired.

❖ Skipping the Salt—Cooked Pasta Instructions

Instead of adding salt to the water when you boil pasta, as called for on most packages of pasta, skip the salt and instead add 1 tablespoon fresh lemon juice, or ¼ teaspoon crushed dried lemon granules, and ¼ teaspoon mustard powder to the water. It provides great flavor without the sodium.

Easy Chicken Lo Mein

Serves 4	
Per serving:	
Calories:	406.19
Protein:	44.06 g
Carbohydrates:	45.37 g
Total fat:	5.38 g
Sat. fat:	1.35 g
Cholesterol:	96.44 mg
Sodium:	138.59 mg
Fiber:	5.27 g

⅛ teaspoon Minor's Low Sodium Chicken Base
½ cup water
2 (10-ounce) packages Cascadian Farm Organic frozen Chinese Stir-Fry Vegetables
1 tablespoon freeze-dried shallots
1 pound cooked dark and light meat chicken
⅛ cup (or to taste) Mr. Spice Ginger Stir-Fry Sauce

1 pound no-salt-added oat bran pasta
1 teaspoon lemon juice
⅛ teaspoon mustard powder
1 teaspoon cornstarch
¼ teaspoon toasted sesame oil
Optional: 4 thinly sliced scallions
Optional: Bragg Liquid Aminos or low-sodium soy sauce

1. Add the chicken base and water to a large microwave-safe bowl; microwave on high for 30 seconds. Stir to dissolve the base into the water. Add the vegetables and freeze-dried shallots; microwave on high for 3 to 5 minutes. Drain some of the broth into a small nonstick sauté pan and set aside. Add the chicken and stir-fry sauce to the vegetables; stir well. Cover and set aside.

2. Consult the package for the pasta. In a large pot, bring the noted amount of water to a boil, but omit the salt. Add the pasta, lemon juice, and mustard powder.

3. While the pasta cooks, in a small cup or bowl, add a tablespoon of water to the cornstarch and whisk to make a slurry. Bring the reserved broth in the sauté pan to a boil over medium-high heat. Whisk in the slurry; cook for at least 1 minute, stirring constantly.

4. Once the mixture thickens, remove from heat; add the toasted sesame oil to the broth mixture, then whisk again. Pour the thickened broth mixture over the vegetables and chicken; toss to mix. Cover and microwave the chicken-vegetable mixture at 70 percent power for 2 minutes or until the chicken is heated through.

5. Drain the pasta; add it to the chicken-vegetable mixture and stir to combine. Divide among 4 plates. Garnish with chopped scallions and serve with the Bragg Liquid Aminos at the table, if desired.

Three-Cheese English Muffin Pizzas

4 Thomas' English muffins, split
Spectrum Naturals Extra-Virgin
  Olive Spray Oil
½ cup Low-Fat Tomato Sauce
  (page 199)
2 tablespoons, plus 2 teaspoons
  grated Parmesan cheese
Optional: Sliced fresh mushrooms
Optional: Chopped onion or onion
  powder

Optional: Chopped roasted red
  pepper (see instructions for
  roasting peppers on page 58)
Optional: Chopped fresh bell
  pepper
Optional: Minced fresh garlic or
  garlic powder
½ cup shredded Cheddar cheese
½ cup shredded whole-milk moz-
  zarella cheese

Serves 4	
Per serving:	
Calories:	211.90
Protein:	10.19 g
Carbohydrates:	29.36 g
Total fat:	6.09 g
Sat. fat:	3.89 g
Cholesterol:	16.00 mg
Sodium:	368.43 mg
Fiber:	0.58 g

1. Preheat oven to 400°. (For easier cleanup, line a baking sheet with nonstick aluminum foil.)
2. Lightly spray the bottom of each muffin with the spray oil. Top each slice with 1 tablespoon of the tomato sauce. Sprinkle 1 teaspoon of the Parmesan cheese over the sauce. Add choice of optional ingredients, if using. Mix the Cheddar and mozzarella cheese together; top each muffin half with 1 tablespoon of the cheese mixture. Bake for 8 to 10 minutes, until the cheese bubbles.

❖ Appetizer Options

Either English muffin pizza recipe can be used to make 16 a-little-bigger-than-bite-size appetizer servings. Cut each muffin half "pizza" into quarters and arrange on a serving tray.

Crunchy Crust English Muffin Pizzas

Serves 4	
Per serving:	
Calories:	203.11
Protein:	9.80 g
Carbohydrates:	29.42 g
Total fat:	5.26 g
Sat. fat:	3.32 g
Cholesterol:	14.05 mg
Sodium:	350.68 mg
Fiber:	0.58 g

4 Thomas' English muffins, split
Spectrum Naturals Extra-Virgin
    Olive Spray Oil
½ cup Low-Fat Tomato Sauce
    (page 199)
2 tablespoons, plus 2 teaspoons
    grated Parmesan cheese
Optional: Dried red pepper flakes
    or Mrs. Dash Extra-Spicy
    Seasoning Blend, to taste
Optional: Sliced fresh mushrooms

Optional: Chopped onion or onion
    powder
Optional: Chopped roasted red
    pepper (page 58)
Optional: Chopped fresh bell
    pepper
Optional: Minced fresh garlic or
    garlic powder
½ cup shredded Cheddar cheese
½ cup shredded whole-milk moz-
    zarella cheese

1. Toast the English muffin halves, either in the toaster or under the broiler. If toasting under the broiler, first lightly spray both sides of the muffin halves with the spray oil. Place on a baking sheet; toast the bottoms first, then turn the muffins and toast the tops. For easier clean up, line the baking sheet with nonstick aluminum foil. If toasted in the toaster, lightly spray the bottom of each muffin with the spray oil after toasting.
2. Top each slice with 1 tablespoon of tomato sauce. Sprinkle 1 teaspoon of Parmesan cheese over the sauce. Add choice of optional ingredients, if using. Top each muffin half with 1 tablespoon of Cheddar and mozzarella. Place several inches under the broiler for about 3 minutes or until the cheese bubbles.

Tuna-Pasta Salad

1 (6-ounce) can Chicken of the Sea "50% Less Sodium" Tuna, drained

1 tablespoon Hellmann's or Best Foods Real Mayonnaise

1 tablespoon nonfat yogurt

2 teaspoons sweet pickle relish

1 teaspoon cane sugar

1 teaspoon champagne or white wine vinegar

2 cups cooked spaghetti (cooked in unsalted water)

½ cup diced celery

10 medium-size baby carrots, sliced

Optional: ½ teaspoon Spice House Salt-Free Sunny Paris Seasoning

Chopped fresh or freeze-dried chives, scallion, or freeze-dried green onion

Serves 2	
Per serving:	
Calories:	376.31
Protein:	29.82 g
Carbohydrates:	54.75 g
Total fat:	3.72 g
Sat. fat:	0.47 g
Cholesterol:	39.56 mg
Sodium:	305.56 mg
Fiber:	4.26 g

1. Combine the drained tuna, mayonnaise, yogurt, relish, sugar, and vinegar in a bowl; stir until well mixed.

2. Add the cooked spaghetti, the celery, and carrots; toss to mix. Mix in the optional seasoning, if using. Refrigerate until needed. Garnish with chopped chives, scallion, or green onion, if desired.

❋ Tiny Tastes as You Go

Remember: It's easier to adjust seasonings up than it is to subtract them if you add too much. Take a sample nibble before you serve a dish, and adjust the seasonings, if necessary.

Tuna-Fresh Tomato Pizza
Pizza Crust

Serves 4	
Per serving:	
Calories:	124.35
Protein:	3.61 g
Carbohydrates:	24.49 g
Total fat:	1.10 g
Sat. fat:	0.16 g
Cholesterol:	0.00 mg
Sodium:	73.80 mg
Fiber:	1.05 g

1 cup warm water
¼ teaspoon granulated sugar
1 teaspoon active dry yeast

1 teaspoon olive oil
1 cup unbleached all-purpose flour
Optional: ½ teaspoon sea salt

1. Mix the water, sugar, and yeast together in a small bowl and set aside for 5 to 10 minutes to allow the yeast to proof.
2. Once the yeast is bubbling, add to it the olive oil, flour, and sea salt. Stir together with a fork, working the dough until it pulls away from the side of the bowl. It's important that the dough be worked enough to form a ball in the bowl; however, it will still be very sticky.
3. Turn the dough out onto a lightly floured surface and, using a knife or pastry cutter, divide it into 4 sections. Next, oil your hands by rubbing ¼ teaspoon of olive oil over your palms. (The Nutritional Analysis for this recipe was done assuming you'd oil your hands more than once. Odds are that you won't have to do that, so the actual fat content will be somewhat less than given.) Shape each of the 4 dough sections into a ball, then 1 by 1, flatten each ball until it forms a "crust" about 6" in diameter. Place each crust on a jelly roll baking sheet treated with nonstick spray. At that size, you should be able to arrange all 4 crusts onto 1 sheet. Using the tongs of a fork, prick each crust a few times. (This prevents them from rising too high during baking and creating pita-style bread instead.)

❀ It Only Takes a Tad
A pinch of sugar is a wonderful flavor enhancer and helps cut the acidity in cooked tomato sauces and soups.

Tuna-Fresh Tomato Pizza
Pizza Topping

2 medium-size tomatoes
½ teaspoon garlic powder
½ teaspoon dried basil
¼ teaspoon dried parsley
⅛ teaspoon dried oregano
1 (6-ounce) can Chicken of the
  Sea "50% Less Sodium" Tuna,
  drained

1 cup nonfat cottage cheese
1 teaspoon Ener-G Potato Flour
4 teaspoons grated Parmesan
  cheese

Serves 4	
Per serving:	
Calories:	91.80
Protein:	15.66 g
Carbohydrates:	4.28 g
Total fat:	1.17 g
Sat. fat:	0.45 g
Cholesterol:	22.60 mg
Sodium:	119.86 mg
Fiber:	0.73 g

1. Preheat oven to 400°.
2. Clean and peel the tomatoes. Slice or dice them and arrange them evenly over the pizza crusts. Combine the garlic powder, basil, parsley, and oregano; sprinkle over the tomatoes. Spread the drained tuna over the pizzas.
3. Mix together the cottage cheese, potato flour, and Parmesan cheese in a bowl, then divide evenly over the pizzas.
4. Bake until the cheese bubbles and the crusts are done. The amount of baking time—anywhere from 3 to 8 minutes or more—will vary considerably, depending on how thin you've made your crusts, which affects how thick you've topped those crusts. (Prebaked crusts will also take less time.)

❁ Leveraging Lycopene

There's evidence that the nutritional benefits of tomatoes increase when you cook them, because cooking makes lycopene more available to the body than when tomatoes are eaten raw. Lycopene is the antioxidant that gives tomatoes their red color; recent studies indicate lycopene helps lessen the chance of certain cancers.

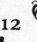

Breads

Basic White Bread

Serves 24	
Per serving:	
Calories:	86.95
Protein:	2.22 g
Carbohydrates:	16.14 g
Total fat:	1.34 g
Sat. fat:	0.19 g
Cholesterol:	0.00 mg
Sodium:	97.40 mg
Fiber:	0.60 g

1 teaspoon active dry yeast
1 teaspoon granulated sugar
1⅓ cups lukewarm water
  (about 105°)

2 tablespoons extra-virgin olive oil
1 teaspoon fine sea salt
4 cups unbleached bread flour

1. To make the dough: In the bowl of a heavy-duty electric mixer fitted with a dough-hook attachment, combine the yeast, sugar, and water. Mix on lowest speed to blend. Let stand until the yeast bubbles, about 5 minutes.

2. Add the oil and salt; mix on lowest speed to blend. Add 3 cups of the flour and resume mixing at the lowest speed, adding the remaining flour a little at a time until the flour has been absorbed and the dough forms a ball and pulls away from the side of the mixer. (Humidity and other factors can affect how much flour is used, so more or less may be needed. If it takes more, continue to add flour 1 tablespoon at a time until you get the described results.) Increase mixer to the speed recommended by the manufacturer for kneading dough; mix until the dough is soft and has a satiny sheen, about 4 to 5 minutes.

3. Transfer the dough to a bowl that has a capacity of 3 times the size of the ball of dough; cover tightly with plastic wrap and place in the refrigerator. Let the dough rise in the refrigerator until doubled or tripled in bulk, 8 to 12 hours. The dough can be kept for 2 to 3 days in the refrigerator. Simply punch down the dough as it doubles or triples.

4. To bake the bread: Treat a bread pan with olive oil or nonstick cooking spray. Remove the dough from the refrigerator and punch down. If necessary, rub a little olive oil on your hands and work the dough by folding it over itself a few times, pinching the resulting "seam" together. Arrange in the pan, seam-side down. Brush a little oil over the top of the dough. Cover with a cotton towel and set in a warm place and let the dough rise until doubled in size. Preheat oven to 350°.

5. Cut 1 or 2 slits in the top of the dough. Bake for 30 to 40 minutes, or until the bread has a hollow sound when "thumped." Let cool in the pan for a few minutes, then remove from the pan and cool on a wire rack.

Savory Beer Bread

¾ cup warm beer
2 teaspoons active dry yeast
1 tablespoon granulated sugar
2¼ cups unbleached all-purpose
   flour
½ cup oat bran or rye flour
¼ teaspoon salt
¼ cup walnut or other cold-pressed
   oil, plus extra for greasing

½ cup minced sweet onion
¼ cup, plus 2 tablespoons walnuts, coarsely chopped
1 small egg, beaten
1 teaspoon water
Optional: Fresh or dried rosemary

Serves 24	
Per serving:	
Calories:	85.33
Protein:	2.12 g
Carbohydrates:	11.64 g
Total fat:	3.51 g
Sat. fat:	0.38 g
Cholesterol:	6.55 mg
Sodium:	27.15 mg
Fiber:	0.85 g

1. In a microwave-safe measuring cup, heat the beer to lukewarm (105° to 115°), about 20 to 30 seconds in the microwave on high. Add the yeast and sugar; let stand for 10 minutes or until the yeast begins to bubble.

2. Combine the flour, oat bran, and salt in a large bowl. Make a well in the center. Pour the yeast mixture and oil into the well; stir until blended. The dough should form a ball and easily pull away from the bowl. If not, add more flour 1 tablespoon at a time.

3. Turn the dough out onto a floured surface. Sprinkle flour over the top of the dough and pat some onto your hands. Knead the dough by pressing it against the floured surface with the heels of your hands, then fold it back onto itself. Knead until the dough is glossy, smooth, and elastic, about 10 minutes.

4. Grease a large bowl with walnut or other cold-pressed oil. Place the kneaded dough in the bowl and turn to coat with oil. Cover with a damp cotton towel and let rise in a warm place until doubled in size, about 1 hour. (Alternatively, you can cover the bowl with plastic wrap and let the dough rise overnight in the refrigerator. If you do, allow the dough to come to room temperature before you proceed with the next step.)

5. Punch down the dough; add the onion and walnuts, and knead into the dough until evenly distributed throughout.

6. Preheat oven to 375°.

(continues on page 214)

Savory Beer Bread (continued)

7. Turn the dough out onto a floured surface. Divide the dough into thirds. Using your hands, roll each of the pieces into 12"-long ropes. Braid 3 ropes together to form a loaf. Tuck the ends under and place on an 18" × 12" baking sheet. Cover with a cotton towel and let rise until doubled in bulk, about 45 minutes to 1 hour. In a small bowl, beat together the egg and water. Brush the tops of the loaf with the egg wash and sprinkle with rosemary, if desired. Bake for 45 to 50 minutes or until crusty and brown. (The bread should sound hollow when you thump it with your fingers.) Cool on the pan for 10 minutes. Turn out onto a wire rack to cool completely. Slice with a serrated bread knife.

Bread Machine White Bread

Serves 24	
Per serving:	
Calories:	86.14
Protein:	2.82 g
Carbohydrates:	17.34 g
Total fat:	0.43 g
Sat. fat:	0.08 g
Cholesterol:	0.32 mg
Sodium:	57.62 mg
Fiber:	0.62 g

1¼ cups skim milk
1 tablespoon light olive, canola, or other cold-pressed vegetable oil
½ teaspoon salt
2 tablespoons nonfat milk powder

4 cups unbleached all-purpose or bread flour
1 tablespoon granulated sugar
2½ teaspoons active dry yeast

Use the light-crust setting on your bread machine, and add the ingredients to your bread machine in the order recommended by the manufacturer (which is usually in the order given here), being careful that the yeast doesn't come in contact with the salt.

Old-Style Whole-Wheat Bread

1 cup warm water
1¼ teaspoons active dry yeast
1½ cups unbleached all-purpose or
   bread flour
1 tablespoon granulated sugar
¼ cup hot water
¼ teaspoon salt
⅛ teaspoon mustard powder

Pinch dried lemon granules,
   crushed
¼ cup brown sugar
1½ tablespoons Spectrum Naturals
   Organic All-Vegetable Shortening
1½ cups whole-wheat flour

Serves 20	
Per serving:	
Calories:	86.18
Protein:	2.27 g
Carbohydrates:	17.06 g
Total fat:	1.24 g
Sat. fat:	0.49 g
Cholesterol:	0.00 mg
Sodium:	30.87 mg
Fiber:	1.39 g

1. Add the yeast to the warm water. Stir in the all-purpose flour and
   granulated sugar. Beat the mixture until smooth, either by hand or
   with a mixer. Set the mixture in a warm place to "proof" until it
   becomes foamy and bubbly (up to 1 hour).
2. Combine the hot water, salt, mustard powder, lemon granules, brown
   sugar, and shortening; stir. Allow to cool until lukewarm. (Stirring until
   the brown sugar dissolves should be sufficient to cool the water; test
   to be sure, because adding liquid that's too warm can "kill" the yeast.)
   Add to the bubbly flour mixture (the "sponge"). Stir in the whole-
   wheat flour and beat until smooth, but *do not knead*.
3. Divide the dough into 2 loaf pans treated with nonstick spray; cover
   and set in a warm place until doubled in size. Preheat oven to 350°
   and bake for 50 minutes.

❊ Feeding the Yeast
*Bread recipes need some sugar or sweetener, such as honey, to
"feed" the yeast. This helps the yeast work, which in turn helps
the bread rise.*

French Bread

2½ teaspoons active dry yeast	2 cups unbleached all-purpose flour
2½ cups warm water	¼ teaspoon salt
2 cups unbleached bread flour	Optional: Cornmeal

Serves 24	
Per serving:	
Calories:	77.06
Protein:	2.31 g
Carbohydrates:	16.06 g
Total fat:	0.22 g
Sat. fat:	0.03 g
Cholesterol:	0.00 mg
Sodium:	24.85 mg
Fiber:	0.65 g

1. Add the yeast to the water; stir to dissolve. Set aside for 5 to 10 minutes, until the yeast is bubbling to the top. Add the flours and salt to a mixing bowl. If using an electric mixer, use the dough hook and mix on low to combine. Pour in the yeast-water mixture. Mix on low until combined; the dough should form a ball and pull away from the side of the bowl.

2. Add more water or flour, if necessary. If your mixer can handle this much dough, knead at medium-high speed for 5 minutes or until the dough is glossy and elastic. (You should be able to pull the dough gently without it sticking to your fingers.) Otherwise, knead by hand for about 15 minutes by pressing it against the floured surface with the heels of your hands, then folding it back onto itself.

3. Form the dough into a round and cover with a bowl turned upside down over the top. Let rise for 2 hours. Punch down, cover, and let rise for another 1½ hours. Punch down again and divide the dough in half. Roll each half into an elongated loaf. Place on a heavy baking pan treated with nonstick spray or dusted with cornmeal. Use a sharp knife to cut several vents into the top of each loaf. Cover with a damp cotton towel and let rise until doubled.

4. As the loaves rise, place 1 shelf so that it's in the lower third of the oven and the top shelf so it's in the upper third. Preheat oven to 450°. Place a pan of hot water on the bottom shelf; also have a mister filled with water at the ready.

5. Remove the cotton towel covering the loaves and place the baking sheet with risen bread loaves in the oven. Quickly mist water across the tops of the loaves. (This creates an immediate rush of steam and helps form a good crust.) Bake for 25 minutes or until the loaves are nicely browned and have a hollow sound when "thumped" on the bottom crust.

Bread Machine Honey Whole-Wheat Bread

Serves 24	
Per serving:	
Calories:	87.47
Protein:	3.27 g
Carbohydrates:	16.91 g
Total fat:	0.75 g
Sat. fat:	0.17 g
Cholesterol:	9.48 mg
Sodium:	61.23 mg
Fiber:	1.06 g

1¼ cups skim milk
1 tablespoon light olive, canola, or other cold-pressed vegetable oil
1 large egg, beaten
¼ cup oat bran
2 tablespoons nonfat buttermilk powder
½ teaspoon salt
3 cups unbleached all-purpose or bread flour
¾ cup whole-wheat flour
1 tablespoon honey
2½ teaspoons active dry yeast

Check the manufacturer's manual for whole-grain bread settings; otherwise, use the light-crust setting. Add the ingredients to your bread machine in the order recommended by the manufacturer (which is usually in the order given here), being careful that the yeast doesn't come in contact with the salt.

Raised Buttermilk Biscuits

Serves 24	
Per serving:	
Calories:	91.14
Protein:	1.78 g
Carbohydrates:	11.56 g
Total fat:	4.30 g
Sat. fat:	2.26 g
Cholesterol:	5.48 mg
Sodium:	33.10 mg
Fiber:	0.44 g

¾ cup cultured lowfat buttermilk, warm
⅛ cup granulated sugar
2½ teaspoons active dry yeast
2½ cups unbleached all-purpose flour
¼ teaspoon salt
½ teaspoon low-salt baking powder
¼ cup unsalted butter
¼ cup Spectrum Naturals Organic All-Vegetable Shortening

1. Put the buttermilk and sugar in a food processor and process until mixed. Sprinkle the yeast over the buttermilk-sugar mixture and pulse once or twice to mix. Allow the mixture to sit at room temperature for about 5 minutes or until the yeast begins to work and is bubbling. Add the remaining ingredients to the food processor and pulse until mixed, being careful not to overprocess the dough.
2. Preheat oven to 400°. Drop by heaping teaspoon per biscuit onto a baking sheet treated with nonstick spray. Set the tray in a warm place and allow the biscuits to rise for about 15 minutes. Bake for 12 to 15 minutes.

Bread Machine 7-Grain Bread

Serves 24	
Per serving:	
Calories:	79.54
Protein:	3.05 g
Carbohydrates:	15.30 g
Total fat:	0.79 g
Sat. fat:	0.17 g
Cholesterol:	9.17 mg
Sodium:	60.35 mg
Fiber:	1.22 g

1¼ cups skim milk
2 tablespoons nonfat milk powder
1 tablespoon extra-light olive or canola oil
¾ cup dry 7-grain cereal
½ cup oat bran
¼ teaspoon sea salt
⅛ teaspoon dried lemon granules, crushed
Pinch mustard powder
2¼ cups unbleached all-purpose or bread flour
½ cup whole-wheat flour
1 tablespoon honey
2½ teaspoons active dry yeast

Add the ingredients to your bread machine in the order recommended by the manufacturer (which is usually in the order given here), being careful that the yeast doesn't come in contact with the salt. Bake on whole-wheat bread setting.

Bread Machine Cheesy Cornbread

Serves 24	
Per serving:	
Calories:	100.71
Protein:	3.08 g
Carbohydrates:	15.93 g
Total fat:	2.64 g
Sat. fat:	0.69 g
Cholesterol:	2.89 mg
Sodium:	50.03 mg
Fiber:	0.85 g

1¼ cups water
¼ cup dried nonfat milk powder
1 tablespoon honey
2 tablespoons, plus 2 teaspoons canola oil
1 teaspoon natural butter flavoring
2½ teaspoons active dry yeast
2½ cups bread flour
1 cup yellow cornmeal
¼ teaspoon mustard powder
¼ teaspoon sea salt
⅛ teaspoon dried lemon granules, crushed
½ cup grated Cheddar cheese
1 tablespoon grated Parmesan cheese

Bring the water to just below the boiling point; remove from heat. Immediately whisk in the milk powder, honey, oil, and butter flavoring; let cool to room temperature. Add the ingredients *except* the Cheddar and Parmesan cheese in the order suggested by your bread machine manual, and process on the basic bread cycle. At the beeper (or at the end of the first kneading), add the cheeses.

Bread Machine Oat Bran Bread

¼ cup water
1 cup nonfat cottage cheese
2 tablespoons unsalted butter
1 large egg
1 tablespoon granulated sugar
¼ teaspoon baking soda
¼ teaspoon salt
⅛ teaspoon dried lemon granules, crushed
2¾ cups bread flour
¼ cup oat bran
2½ teaspoons active dry yeast

Serves 24	
Per serving:	
Calories:	72.66
Protein:	2.98 g
Carbohydrates:	11.96 g
Total fat:	1.37 g
Sat. fat:	0.71 g
Cholesterol:	11.87 mg
Sodium:	41.33 mg
Fiber:	0.51 g

1. Add the ingredients to your bread machine in the order recommended by the manufacturer (which is usually in the order given here), being careful that the yeast doesn't come in contact with the salt.
2. Check the bread machine at the "beep" to make sure the dough is pulling away from the sides of the pan and forming a ball. Add water or flour, if needed. (You do not want the dough to be overly dry.)
3. Bake at the white bread setting, light crust.

Bread Machine New York Rye

1⅛ cups water
2 tablespoons honey
¼ teaspoon salt
⅛ teaspoon mustard powder
⅛ teaspoon dried lemon granules, crushed
4 teaspoons olive or canola oil
1 large egg, beaten
¼ cup dried nonfat milk powder
1 tablespoon caraway seeds
2½ cups bread flour
1¼ cups rye flour
¼ cup whole-wheat flour
¼ cup oat bran
2½ teaspoons active dry yeast

Serves 24	
Per serving:	
Calories:	93.54
Protein:	2.78 g
Carbohydrates:	17.72 g
Total fat:	1.31 g
Sat. fat:	0.22 g
Cholesterol:	8.98 mg
Sodium:	31.47 mg
Fiber:	1.57 g

1. Add the ingredients in the order suggested by your bread machine manual and process on the basic bread cycle according to the manufacturer's directions.
2. Bake at the white bread setting, light crust.

Buttery Batter Biscuits

Serves 24	
Per serving:	
Calories:	98.41
Protein:	2.19 g
Carbohydrates:	12.96 g
Total fat:	4.15 g
Sat. fat:	2.51 g
Cholesterol:	10.90 mg
Sodium:	132.15 mg
Fiber:	0.42 g

3 cups unbleached all-purpose flour
¼ teaspoon salt
1½ teaspoons baking soda
1 tablespoon cream of tartar
1 teaspoon baking powder
½ cup unsalted butter
1⅓ cups 1% milk

1. Preheat oven to 400°. For quick mixing, use a food processor. Just add all of the ingredients at once and pulse until just blended. Be careful not to overprocess this dough; if you do, the rolls won't be as light.
2. To mix by hand, sift together the dry ingredients, then cut in the butter using a pastry blender or fork until the mixture resembles coarse crumbs. Add the milk and stir until the mixture pulls away from the sides of the bowl.
3. Use 1 heaping tablespoon for each biscuit, dropping the dough onto baking sheets treated with nonstick spray. (You can also use pan liners, such as parchment or nonstick aluminum foil.) Bake until golden brown, about 20 to 30 minutes.

✿ Heathful Fat Facts

Most commercial bread not only contain lots of preservatives (most of which aren't even listed on the label), they also usually use shortening, which contains hydrogenated oil, a less healthy fat choice. You can substitute olive or other cold-pressed vegetable oil—like canola—for the butter in any bread recipe. This will significantly reduce the overall amount of saturated fat. If you use butter, be sure to use unsalted; otherwise, the bread will be higher in sodium, plus the higher moisture content of salted butter can affect the amount of flour needed to produce a good texture.

Lemon Pear Scones

1 cup oatmeal or oat bran, or a
½ cup of each
1 cup unbleached all-purpose flour
⅓ cup, plus 2 tablespoons granulated sugar
1½ teaspoons low-salt baking
powder
½ teaspoon baking soda
1 teaspoon dried ground ginger
¼ teaspoon cinnamon
¼ teaspoon nutmeg

Pinch salt
2 teaspoons lemon zest
3 tablespoons unsalted butter,
cut into small pieces
⅔ cup plain nonfat yogurt
1 large egg, lightly beaten
1 teaspoon vanilla extract
2 teaspoons lemon extract
½ cup peeled and grated pear

Serves 12	
Per serving:	
Calories:	143.49
Protein:	3.62 g
Carbohydrates:	23.70 g
Total fat:	4.01 g
Sat. fat:	2.05 g
Cholesterol:	25.67 mg
Sodium:	66.54 mg
Fiber:	1.41 g

1. Preheat oven to 400°. Treat a baking sheet or jelly roll pan with nonstick cooking spray.
2. In a large bowl, combine the oatmeal, flour, ⅓ cup of the sugar, baking powder, baking soda, ginger, cinnamon, nutmeg, salt, and lemon zest; mix well. Cut in the butter until crumbly.
3. In a separate bowl, mix together the yogurt, beaten egg, vanilla extract, and lemon extract. Add to the dry ingredients, using a fork to mix the wet ingredients in to moisten the dry. Fold in the grated pear.
4. Drop ¼ cupfuls of batter in semiflattened mounds on the treated baking sheet. Sprinkle with the remaining sugar. Bake for 16 to 18 minutes, until light golden brown. Serve warm.

❈ Teatime Tip
You can underbake some of the scones and then, once they've cooled, wrap them in nonstick foil and freeze them until needed. When needed, pop the foil-wrapped scones into a preheated 350° oven for 15 to 20 minutes.

Bread Machine Potato Water Sourdough Oat Bran Bread

Serves 24	
Per serving:	
Calories:	82.61
Protein:	2.82 g
Carbohydrates:	16.82 g
Total fat:	0.80 g
Sat. fat:	0.14 g
Cholesterol:	0.20 mg
Sodium:	54.37 mg
Fiber:	0.99 g

1 cup nonfat milk
½ cup Potato Water Sourdough
  Starter (see recipe following)
2 tablespoons extra-virgin olive oil
¾ cup oat bran

3¼ cups unbleached all-purpose
  flour
½ teaspoon salt
2 teaspoons granulated sugar
1 teaspoon active dry yeast

1. Add the ingredients to your bread machine in the order recommended by the manufacturer (which is usually in the order given here), being careful that the yeast doesn't come in contact with the salt. Set the bread maker at the white bread setting, light crust.
2. Check the bread machine at the "beep" to make sure the dough is pulling away from the sides of the pan and forming a ball. Add water or flour, if needed. (You do not want the dough to be overly dry.)

Potato Water Sourdough Starter

1 cup potato water (water drained
  off of unsalted boiled potatoes)
¾ cup unbleached all-purpose flour

1 teaspoon granulated sugar
1 teaspoon active dry yeast
¾ teaspoon sea salt

1. Combine all the ingredients in a glass container (such as a mayonnaise jar) and cover the jar with cheesecloth.
2. Allow to sit at room temperature, stirring the mixture or jiggling the jar occasionally to keep it mixed. (The length of time you leave the dough starter at room temperature will depend on how sour you like your bread. If you prefer a milder flavor, only allow the starter to sit for 6 hours. You can leave the starter at room temperature for up to 2 days.)
3. Store the starter in the refrigerator in a container with a small hole in the lid; the hole allows the gasses to escape. Replenish the starter as needed with equal parts water and flour.

Bread Machine Awesome Orange Bread

1 large egg
¼ cup Cascadian Farm Frozen
   Organic Orange Juice Concentrate
1 cup water
2 tablespoons canola oil
1 teaspoon vanilla extract
1 teaspoon orange zest
½ teaspoon lemon zest
¼ teaspoon dried ground ginger
Pinch cinnamon

Pinch cloves
Pinch nutmeg
¼ teaspoon salt
⅛ cup oat bran
1½ cups unbleached bread flour
2¼ cups unbleached all-purpose
   flour
⅛ cup granulated sugar
2 tablespoons dried nonfat milk
2½ teaspoons active dry yeast

Serves 24	
Per serving:	
Calories:	90.97
Protein:	2.59 g
Carbohydrates:	16.44 g
Total fat:	1.61 g
Sat. fat:	0.19 g
Cholesterol:	8.98 mg
Sodium:	30.79 mg
Fiber:	0.65 g

Unless the instructions for your bread machine differ, add the ingredients in the order listed here. Use the light-crust setting.

Bread Machine Honey 7-Grain Bread

1¼ cups skim milk
2 tablespoons nonfat milk powder
1 tablespoon canola oil
¾ cup dry 7-grain cereal
½ cup oat bran
⅛ teaspoon dried lemon granules,
   crushed
Pinch cinnamon

Pinch nutmeg
¼ teaspoon salt
2¼ cups unbleached all-purpose or
   bread flour
½ cup whole-wheat flour
1 tablespoon honey
2½ teaspoons active dry yeast

Serves 24	
Per serving:	
Calories:	79.17
Protein:	3.02 g
Carbohydrates:	15.30 g
Total fat:	0.77 g
Sat. fat:	0.16 g
Cholesterol:	8.11 mg
Sodium:	35.81 mg
Fiber:	1.22 g

Add the ingredients to your bread machine in the order recommended by the manufacturer (which is usually in the order given here), being careful that the yeast doesn't come in contact with the salt. Bake on whole-wheat bread setting.

Bread Machine Reduced-Sodium Hawaiian-Style Bread

Serves 24	
Per serving:	
Calories:	93.83
Protein:	2.50 g
Carbohydrates:	17.16 g
Total fat:	1.57 g
Sat. fat:	0.18 g
Cholesterol:	8.98 mg
Sodium:	30.78 mg
Fiber:	0.58 g

1 large egg
½ cup unsweetened pineapple juice
¾ cup water
2 tablespoons canola oil
1 teaspoon vanilla extract
1 teaspoon orange zest
½ teaspoon lemon zest
½ teaspoon dried ground ginger

¼ teaspoon salt
1½ cups unbleached bread flour
2¼ cups unbleached all-purpose flour
¼ cup granulated sugar
2 tablespoons dried nonfat milk
2½ teaspoons active dry yeast

Unless the instructions for your bread machine differ, add the ingredients in the order listed here. Bake on the light-crust setting.

Bread Machine Cottage Cheese Bread

Serves 24	
Per serving:	
Calories:	78.32
Protein:	3.03 g
Carbohydrates:	12.70 g
Total fat:	1.57 g
Sat. fat:	0.19 g
Cholesterol:	9.28 mg
Sodium:	41.21 mg
Fiber:	0.48 g

¼ cup water
1 cup nonfat cottage cheese
2 tablespoons canola oil
1 large egg
1 tablespoon granulated sugar
¼ teaspoon baking soda

Pinch nutmeg
⅛ teaspoon dried lemon granules, crushed
¼ teaspoon salt
3 cups bread flour
2½ teaspoons active dry yeast

1. Add the ingredients to your bread machine in the order recommended by the manufacturer (which is usually in the order given here), being careful that the yeast doesn't come in contact with the salt.
2. Check the bread machine at the "beep" to make sure the dough is pulling away from the sides of the pan and forming a ball. Add water or flour, if needed. (You do not want the dough to be overly dry.) Bake at the white bread setting, light crust.

Flour Tortillas

2 cups unbleached all-purpose
  flour
¼ teaspoon salt
1 teaspoon low-salt baking powder

1 tablespoon lard
¾ cup cold water

Serves 12	
Per serving:	
Calories:	85.86
Protein:	2.15 g
Carbohydrates:	16.09 g
Total fat:	1.27 g
Sat. fat:	0.45 g
Cholesterol:	1.01 mg
Sodium:	49.24 mg
Fiber:	0.57 g

1. Thoroughly mix the dry ingredients in a bowl. Use a pastry blender or fork to cut in the lard and enough water to make a stiff dough. Divide into 12 balls.
2. Roll out on a lightly floured board, making them as thin as possible. Bring a griddle or nonstick pan treated with nonstick spray to temperature over medium heat. Cook the tortillas by placing them on griddle or in pan 1 at a time. Turn the tortillas when the top side begins to show some puffiness or blisters; turn and cook until the other side is lightly browned. (Total cooking time will be about 2 minutes per tortilla.)

✿ Grilled Tortillas

Tortillas can also be "baked" on an outdoor grill over indirect heat; as you would for grilling pizza crust, just make sure the grids are clean and well-seasoned so that the dough doesn't stick.

Corn Tortillas

2 cups masa harina
¼ teaspoon salt
¼ teaspoon mustard powder

2 tablespoons lard
1¼ cups warm water

Serves 16	
Per serving:	
Calories:	66.44
Protein:	1.33 g
Carbohydrates:	10.87 g
Total fat:	2.14 g
Sat. fat:	0.70 g
Cholesterol:	1.52 mg
Sodium:	37.05 mg
Fiber:	1.37 g

1. Add the masa harina, salt, and mustard powder to a large bowl; mix well. Add the lard and warm water. Use your fingers to work the mixture into a soft dough. Knead the dough until it is no longer sticky. Divide the dough into 16 balls; cover with a cotton towel and let rest for 20 minutes at room temperature.
2. To use a tortilla press, place a small square of wax paper on the bottom part of the open press. Place a corn tortilla ball almost on the center of the wax paper—a little more toward the hinge of the press than the handle. Place a second wax paper square on top of the ball and press to flatten slightly. Close the press firmly until the tortilla measures about 6" in diameter. Alternately, roll the tortillas by hand: Flatten each ball between 2 pieces of wax paper and roll out with a rolling pin; or place each ball on a lightly floured surface, dust the top of the ball with some flour, and roll out with a rolling pin. (Try to use as little flour as possible.)
3. Place the tortilla on a moderately hot griddle treated with nonstick spray. Quickly, the edges of the tortilla will begin to dry out. At this point, turn the tortilla. Allow the second side to cook for a slightly longer period until it is slightly browned. Flip it back onto the first side and let it finish cooking. Allow about 2 minutes total cooking time per tortilla.

❈ Tortilla Tip
You can use a mixer with a dough hook or a food processor to mix corn tortilla dough. Like bread, the dough needs to be kneaded until it's no longer sticky. One southwestern cook says she kneads the dough for 3 minutes when she mixes flour tortillas using her Bosch mixer; those 3 minutes would be about the equivalent of about 10 to 15 minutes of heavy-duty hand kneading.

Thin Flour Tortillas

2 cups unbleached all-purpose flour
1 teaspoon low-salt baking powder
1 tablespoon Spectrum Naturals
   Organic All-Vegetable Shortening

¼ teaspoon salt
¾ cup cold water

Serves 24	
Per serving:	
Calories:	42.93
Protein:	1.08 g
Carbohydrates:	8.05 g
Total fat:	0.64 g
Sat. fat:	0.23 g
Cholesterol:	0.51 mg
Sodium:	24.62 mg
Fiber:	0.29 g

1. Thoroughly mix the flour and baking powder together in a bowl. Using your fingers, rub the shortening into the flour. Dissolve the salt in the water and add it to the flour mixture. Use your fingers to knead the water and flour mixture into a dough, kneading for about 3 minutes. Cover the bowl with a cotton towel; let the dough rest for at least 2 hours. (Do not refrigerate.)

2. After the dough has rested, knead it again. Divide the dough into 24 balls, each about 1½" in diameter. Cover with a cotton towel until needed.

3. To prepare the tortillas, dust your hands with flour. Flatten 1 of the tortilla dough balls between your hands. Transfer to a lightly floured surface and use a rolling pin to roll it into a 7"-diameter round. As you roll the dough, turning it occasionally as you apply the rolling pin helps keep it round.

4. Bring a griddle or nonstick skillet to temperature over medium heat. Place the rolled tortilla on the griddle or in the skillet. (The cooking surface should be hot enough that there is a slight sizzling sound when the dough hits the surface.) Cook for about 20 seconds or until bubbles appear on the surface and the underside is speckled with dark brown. (If it puffs up, use a heat-safe spatula to press it down.) Turn the tortilla; cook it for a slightly shorter time on the other side.

❀ Storing Tortillas

Flour or corn tortillas can be stored flat for several days in the refrigerator, or frozen. There is no need to defrost them before reheating.

Indian Spiced Flatbread

Serves 6	
Per serving:	
Calories:	399.43
Protein:	13.50 g
Carbohydrates:	69.57 g
Total fat:	7.01 g
Sat. fat:	0.86 g
Cholesterol:	36.46 mg
Sodium:	48.54 mg
Fiber:	3.06 g

⅔ cup warm skim milk
1 teaspoon granulated sugar
5 teaspoons active dry yeast
4 cups unbleached all-purpose flour
1 teaspoon baking powder
⅛ teaspoon mustard powder
⅛ teaspoon dried lemon granules,
  crushed
1 teaspoon fennel seeds

2 teaspoons charnushka
1 teaspoon cumin seeds
2 tablespoons canola oil
⅔ cup plain nonfat yogurt
1 large egg, beaten
Spectrum Naturals Canola Spray
  Oil with Butter Flavor
2 teaspoons poppy seeds

1. In a microwave-safe measuring cup, heat the milk until warm (15 to 20 seconds on high). Stir in the sugar and yeast. Set aside for 5 minutes for the yeast to proof.
2. Add the flour, baking powder, mustard powder, lemon granules, fennel seeds, charnushka, and cumin seeds to mixing bowl. Place a cover over the bowl and mix on low with the dough hook long enough to combine the ingredients. Add the milk-yeast mixture, oil, yogurt, and egg. Mix on low until the dough begins to form a ball and pull away from the sides of the bowl, then knead until the mixture becomes elastic. Cover and let the mixture rise until doubled.
3. Place a heavy baking sheet in the oven; preheat oven to 475°.
4. Turn out the dough onto a lightly floured surface. Punch down, then knead the dough for about 1 minute. Divide into 6 equal pieces; cover with a damp cotton towel and let rest for 15 minutes.
5. Roll each naan (flatbread) out to a teardrop (rather than round) shape, leaving the dough about 10 times the thickness of a tortilla or about half the height of a hamburger bun. (Keep the remaining dough covered with the towel while you roll out each naan.) Lightly spray the top of the naan with the spray oil and sprinkle ⅓ teaspoon poppy seeds over the top. Transfer to the baking pan. Bake for 3 minutes,

until puffed, then place under the broiler until the top is lightly browned. Repeat with the remaining 5 naan segments. (If you prefer, you can bake the flatbreads 2 at a time.) The bread is best served warm, immediately after baking; however, it can be baked and then broiled later immediately before serving.

6. If preparing on the grill, grill over indirect heat until puffy, then turn the bread and grill an additional 15 to 30 seconds. Transfer to a plate. Treat the side of the bread that is brownest with the spray oil, sprinkle with the poppy seeds, and return to the grill—poppy seed–side up—for another 15 to 30 seconds.

❈ Pan Quality Affects Baking Time

The quality of your bread pan (bread takes less time to bake in a heavier, steel-clad pan than it does in a lighter aluminum pan; see Appendix B), the humidity, the type of oven you use and how well it maintains the temperature, and other factors can all affect how bread turns out. Putting a pizza stone (see Appendix B) on a lower oven shelf can help maintain oven temperature, even when you're not baking directly on the stone. Putting a pan of water in the oven or using a mister to spritz in some water immediately after placing a loaf in the oven can also help develop a crispier crust.

Americanized Indian Flatbread

Serves 12	
Per serving:	
Calories:	138.16
Protein:	4.43 g
Carbohydrates:	18.42 g
Total fat:	5.10 g
Sat. fat:	0.64 g
Cholesterol:	35.88 mg
Sodium:	71.71 mg
Fiber:	0.76 g

2 cups bleached flour
½ teaspoon low-salt baking powder
½ teaspoon salt
3 tablespoon skim milk
1 cup plain nonfat yogurt
1 teaspoon granulated sugar
1 teaspoon active dry yeast

3 tablespoons canola or other
   cold-pressed vegetable oil, plus
   extra as needed
1 large egg, lightly beaten
1 egg yolk
Optional: Garlic powder
4 teaspoons sesame seeds

1. Mix together the flour, baking powder, and salt into a large bowl; make a well in the center. Mix together the milk and yogurt; heat to lukewarm temperature in a saucepan on the stovetop or in the microwave. Stir the sugar, yeast, oil, and the whole large egg into the milk mixture; pour into the well in the flour. Stir from the center until mixed to a smooth batter. Turn onto a floured surface; knead for about 15 to 20 minutes. (The dough should be elastic but not sticky; sprinkle with a little flour if the dough is sticky.) Place the dough in a covered bowl and let rise until doubled in size, about 3 to 4 hours at normal room temperature.

2. Punch down the dough and turn out onto a floured surface; divide into 12 pieces. Rub a little oil on your hands. Knead each dough piece lightly, then flatten it between your hands, pulling it into an oval to form a pear shape. Put the formed flatbreads onto baking sheets treated with nonstick spray, cover with damp cloth, and let rise for 15 minutes.

3. While the dough rises, preheat the oven to 450°. Beat the egg yolk and brush it over the tops of the flatbreads. Sprinkle with garlic powder and the sesame seeds. Bake for 8 to 10 minutes, until golden brown.

❋ Brown-and-Serve Flatbread

Create your own brown-and-serve flatbreads. Omit brushing the tops with egg yolk. Prebake them for 3 to 4 minutes; let cool and then store in a plastic bag for 1 or 2 days, or freeze until needed. When needed, spray the tops with spray oil and sprinkle them with sesame seeds, garlic powder, or herb seasoning blend.

CHAPTER 13
Snacks and Desserts

Pizza-Flavored Soy Nuts

Serves 8	
Per serving:	
Calories:	203.36
Protein:	17.81 g
Carbohydrates:	14.65 g
Total fat:	10.21 g
Sat. fat:	1.73 g
Cholesterol:	1.50 mg
Sodium:	36.56 mg
Fiber:	3.59 g

2 cups dried soybeans
8 cups water
Spectrum Naturals Extra-Virgin Olive Spray Oil
1 teaspoon Mrs. Dash Tomato Basil Garlic Seasoning Blend
¼ teaspoon dried oregano
¼ teaspoon onion powder
1 or more (to taste) black peppercorns
Optional: ¼ teaspoon paprika
3 tablespoons grated Parmesan cheese

1. Put dried soybeans in a large bowl and pour the water over them. Cover and let soak overnight.
2. Preheat oven to 200°. Drain the soybeans well and blot dry with a towel. Spread the soybeans in a single layer on a baking sheet treated with the spray oil. Bake for 2 hours, stirring occasionally.
3. Raise oven temperature to 375°. Toast the soybeans for 5 minutes or until they're a deep, golden brown.
4. While the soybeans bake, mix together the seasoning blend, oregano, onion powder, and black peppercorns; process to a fine powder in a spice grinder. Pour into a bowl large enough to hold the toasted soy nuts; stir in the paprika, if using it, and Parmesan cheese.
5. Remove the toasted soybeans from the oven and mist with the spray oil. Add the soybeans to the bowl with the seasonings; toss to mix. Serve warm from the oven or at room temperature. Can be made up to a week in advance if stored in a covered container.

❁ Seasoning Substitutions
Instead of the Mrs. Dash Tomato Basil Garlic Seasoning Blend and oregano, you can substitute a mix of salt-free Italian seasoning or the Spice Hunter Salt-Free Italian Pizza Seasoning, garlic powder, and a little tomato powder.

Microwave Air-Popped Popcorn

Yields 4–16 cups	
Per serving:	
Calories:	30.56
Protein:	0.96 g
Carbohydrates:	6.23 g
Total fat:	0.34 g
Sat. fat:	0.05 g
Cholesterol:	0.00 mg
Sodium:	0.32 mg
Fiber:	1.21 g

¼–1 cup popcorn kernels

1. To "air-pop" popcorn in the microwave, add the popcorn kernels to a brown paper bag large enough to hold the yield. Fold down the top. Spray the bag with water (or wet your hand and tap water onto the sides and bottom of the bag). Microwave on high for 3 minutes, or use the popcorn setting if your microwave has it.
2. If popping a smaller (¼-cup) batch, listen closely. Once you no longer hear popcorn popping every 2 seconds, stop the microwave; otherwise, the already-popped popcorn may burn. (There are almost always some unpopped kernels in each batch.)

Cinnamon-Sweet Popcorn

Serves 4	
Per serving:	
Calories:	42.75
Protein:	0.96 g
Carbohydrates:	9.38 g
Total fat:	0.34 g
Sat. fat:	0.05 g
Cholesterol:	0.00 mg
Sodium:	0.35 mg
Fiber:	1.21 g

Spectrum Naturals Canola Spray Oil with Butter Flavor
4 cups air-popped popcorn
1 tablespoon granulated sugar or Whey Low powder
⅛ teaspoon ground cinnamon
Pinch ground nutmeg
Pinch ground cloves
Pinch ground allspice
⅛ teaspoon dried orange granules, crushed

1. Preheat oven to 300°. Treat a jelly roll pan or baking sheet with the spray oil.
2. Spread the popcorn on the pan and lightly coat with the spray oil. Mix together the remaining ingredients; sprinkle over the popcorn. Lightly coat again with the spray oil, if desired.
3. Bake for 5 minutes. Toss the popcorn and rotate the pan, then bake for an additional 5 minutes. Serve warm or at room temperature.

Party Mix Popcorn

Serves 8	
Per serving:	
Calories:	230.56
Protein:	7.49 g
Carbohydrates:	29.52 g
Total fat:	10.22 g
Sat. fat:	1.49 g
Cholesterol:	0.00 mg
Sodium:	110.69 mg
Fiber:	2.86 g

4 cups air-popped popcorn
8 ounces unsalted pretzels
1 cup unsalted dry-roasted peanuts
Spectrum Naturals Canola Spray
   Oil with Butter Flavor
2 teaspoons Bragg Liquid Aminos
1/2 teaspoon garlic powder
1/4 teaspoon onion powder

1/4 teaspoon salt-free lemon pepper
   or Citrus Pepper (page 278)
1/8 teaspoon dried dill, crushed
1/8 teaspoon mustard powder
1/8 teaspoon dried lemon granules,
   crushed

1. Preheat oven to 300°.
2. Mix together the popcorn, pretzels, and peanuts; spread on a nonstick jelly roll pan or baking sheet treated with the spray oil. Mist the top of the mixture with some additional spray oil and the Liquid Aminos.
3. In a small bowl, mix together the remaining ingredients; sprinkle evenly over the popcorn mixture. Bake for 5 minutes. Toss the popcorn mixture and rotate the pan, then bake for an additional 5 minutes. Serve warm or at room temperature.

❈ Smart Choices

Newman's Own Organics has Unsalted, Baked Pretzel Rounds made from organically certified unbleached wheat and rye flour, brown rice sweetener, barley malt, and sunflower oil. The nutritional analysis for the Party Mix Popcorn recipe was calculated using the stats for generic unsalted pretzels. Be careful when you choose which pretzels to buy; many are made with unhealthy oils that are high in saturated fat. Newman's Own Organics also has Fat-Free & Unsalted (microwave) Pop's Corn that can be substituted for air-popped corn.

Corn Tortilla Crisps

4 Corn Tortillas (page 226)
Spectrum Naturals Extra-Virgin
   Olive Spray Oil

Mrs. Dash Extra Spicy Seasoning
   Blend or lime juice and freshly
   ground pepper or salt

1. Preheat oven to 400°. Lightly spray both sides of the tortillas with the spray oil.
2. Place the tortillas on a heavy baking sheet. Bake for 3 to 5 minutes, until crisp. (Be careful; they'll go from lightly browned to burned in a flash!) Season to taste and break each tortilla into 4 pieces.
3. If you prefer equal-sized pieces, you can cut the tortillas before baking by stacking several together on a cutting board and cutting with a pizza cutter or serrated knife; if you do so, decrease the baking time.

Serves 4	
Per serving:	
Calories:	66.44
Protein:	1.33 g
Carbohydrates:	10.87 g
Total fat:	2.14 g
Sat. fat:	0.70 g
Cholesterol:	1.52 mg
Sodium:	37.05 mg
Fiber:	1.37 g

Fruit Sauce

1 teaspoon ground cinnamon
4 teaspoons Vanilla Sugar
1½ teaspoons rosewater

1½ teaspoons orange flower water
4 teaspoons unsalted butter

In a small microwave-safe bowl, combine the cinnamon, sugar, and flower waters; microwave on high for 30 seconds. Stir until the sugar is dissolved, then whisk in the butter. Serve immediately.

❋ Vanilla Sugar
Put 2 cups of sugar and 1 snipped vanilla bean in a blender or food processor; process until the sugar is fine-ground and the vanilla bean is pulverized. Store in an airtight container in the refrigerator or freezer. Use in baking, or mixed with cinnamon on toast.

Serves 4	
Per serving:	
Calories:	50.16
Protein:	0.04 g
Carbohydrates:	4.20 g
Total fat:	3.84 g
Sat. fat:	2.39 g
Cholesterol:	10.36 mg
Sodium:	0.56 mg
Fiber:	0.00 g

Hidden Surprise Cakes

Serves 12	
Per serving:	
Calories:	124.15
Protein:	3.16 g
Carbohydrates:	23.09 g
Total fat:	2.43 g
Sat. fat:	0.95 g
Cholesterol:	53.31 mg
Sodium:	85.03 mg
Fiber:	0.52 g

1 cup unbleached all-purpose flour
⅛ teaspoon salt
1 teaspoon baking powder
3 large eggs
¾ cup Vanilla Sugar (page 235)
1 tablespoon lemon juice
Optional: ½ teaspoon lemon zest

6 tablespoons hot skim milk
1 (1.2-ounce) package Newman's Own Organics Dark Chocolate Peppermint Cups
1 tablespoon cocoa powder

1. Preheat oven to 350°. Treat a 12-section muffin pan with nonstick spray or line with foil liners.
2. In a small bowl, mix together the flour, salt, and baking powder. Add the eggs to the bowl of a food processor or a mixing bowl; pulse or beat until fluffy and lemon colored. Add the sugar, lemon juice, and the optional lemon zest, if using; pulse or beat to mix. Add the flour mixture; process or mix just enough to blend. Add the hot milk and process or mix until blended.
3. Spoon the batter halfway up the muffin sections in the prepared muffin pan. Cut each peppermint cup into 4 equal pieces. Add 1 piece to each muffin section. Spoon the remaining batter over the top of the candy.
4. Bake for 15 minutes or until the cakes are light golden brown and firm to touch. Dust the tops of the cakes with cocoa. Move to a rack to cool.

❈ Sweet Savvy

Dove Dark Chocolate Promises are sodium-free, while Dove Milk Chocolate Promises have 25 milligrams of sodium per serving. Some premium chocolates are even higher in sodium content. Not all chocolates are created equal, so be sure you check the labels.

Carrot Cupcakes

1½ cups unbleached all-purpose
    flour
1 teaspoon baking powder
1 teaspoon baking soda
2 teaspoons Pumpkin Pie Spice
    (page 275)
1 tablespoon granulated sugar
⅛ cup Cascadian Farm Organic
    Frozen Unsweetened Apple Juice
    Concentrate

3 large eggs
1 teaspoon vanilla extract
¼ cup juice from canned unsweet-
    ened crushed pineapple
3 tablespoons nonfat yogurt
1 cup canned unsweetened crushed
    pineapple, well-drained
1 cup finely shredded carrots
¼ cup seedless raisins
2 tablespoons powdered sugar

Serves 9	
Per serving:	
Calories:	151.15
Protein:	5.13 g
Carbohydrates:	28.10 g
Total fat:	2.02 g
Sat. fat:	0.58 g
Cholesterol:	71.02 mg
Sodium:	227.99 mg
Fiber:	1.32 g

1. Preheat oven to 350°. Treat 9 sections of a 12-section muffin pan with nonstick spray or line with foil liners.
2. Sift together the dry ingredients and spices. Add the sugar, apple juice concentrate, and eggs to the bowl of a mixer or food processor; process until well mixed.
3. Add the vanilla, pineapple liquid, and yogurt; pulse to mix. Stir in the dry ingredients. Fold in the crushed pineapple, shredded carrots, and raisins.
4. Divide the batter between the 9 prepared muffin sections in the muffin pan.
5. Bake for 15 minutes or until the cakes are light golden brown and firm to touch. Move to a rack to cool. Dust the tops of the cakes with the powdered sugar.

❁ Gaze at Some Glaze
If you prefer glazed cupcakes, combine the 2 tablespoons of powdered sugar with some unsweetened pineapple juice or water and drizzle over warm cupcakes.

Virgin Bellini

Serves 4	
Per serving:	
Calories:	49.72
Protein:	0.57 g
Carbohydrates:	13.04 g
Total fat:	0.07 g
Sat. fat:	0.01 g
Cholesterol:	0.00 mg
Sodium:	0.21 mg
Fiber:	1.58 g

2 large peaches, peeled, pitted, and cubed
1 tablespoon honey
Optional: Drop of natural almond extract or flavoring or food-grade peppermint oil

Ice cubes
Seltzer water
Optional: Mint sprigs

In a blender or food processor, combine the peaches, honey, and almond extract or flavoring, if using; process until puréed. Divide among 4 champagne flutes or tall glasses filled with ice cubes. Add enough seltzer water to fill the glasses, and stir. Garnish the glasses with fresh mint, if desired. Serve immediately.

Cheddar-Cheesy Apple Nut Muffins

Serves 4	
Per serving:	
Calories:	290.63
Protein:	10.37 g
Carbohydrates:	46.65 g
Total fat:	7.99 g
Sat. fat:	2.60 g
Cholesterol:	7.98 mg
Sodium:	276.45 mg
Fiber:	2.47 g

½ cup plain nonfat yogurt
1 large Granny Smith apple, peeled, cored, and grated
1 tablespoon lemon juice
2 teaspoons honey
⅛ teaspoon ground cinnamon

¼ cup coarse-ground unsalted, dry-roasted almonds
¼ cup shredded Cheddar cheese
4 Thomas' English Muffins, split
Spectrum Naturals Canola Spray Oil with Butter Flavor

Place the yogurt between several layers of paper towels for 10 to 15 minutes. Toss the grated apple with the lemon juice, then place between layers of paper towels and blot dry. Use a spatula to scrape the yogurt and apple into a bowl. Add the honey, cinnamon, almonds, and Cheddar cheese; mix well. Toast the muffins. Lightly spray the tops and bottoms of the muffins with the spray oil. Place the muffin halves (sprayed-sides down) on a baking sheet and top with the Cheddar mixture. Place under the broiler until the cheese is melted and bubbly.

Steamed Raspberry-Lemon Custard

2 large eggs
¼ teaspoon cream of tartar
1 lemon, zested and juiced
¼ teaspoon pure lemon extract
3 tablespoons unbleached all-purpose flour
¼ cup granulated sugar

40 fresh raspberries
Optional: 12 additional fresh raspberries
Optional: 2–4 teaspoons powdered sugar
Optional: Fresh mint leaves

Serves 4	
Per serving:	
Calories:	121.56
Protein:	4.20 g
Carbohydrates:	22.34 g
Total fat:	2.75 g
Sat. fat:	0.80 g
Cholesterol:	106.25 mg
Sodium:	106.95 mg
Fiber:	2.72 g

1. Separate the egg yolks and whites. Add the egg whites to a large bowl and set aside the yolks. Use an electric mixer or wire whisk to beat the egg whites until frothy. Add the cream of tartar; continue to whip or whisk until soft peaks form.

2. In a small bowl, mix together the lemon zest, lemon juice, lemon extract, flour, sugar, and egg yolks; gently fold into the whites with a spatula.

3. Treat 4 (6-ounce) ramekins with nonstick spray. Place 10 raspberries in the bottom of each. Spoon the batter into the ramekins and set them in a steamer with a lid; cover and steam for 15 to 20 minutes.

4. To remove the custards from the ramekins, run a thin knife around edges; turn upside down onto plates. Garnish with raspberries, mint, and a dusting of powdered sugar, if desired.

❀ Steaming Savvy
To steam custards at the same time with other dishes that might affect taste, wrap the ramekins in plastic wrap (so they won't pick up the other aromas) and put them in the top tier of the steamer.

Watermelon Sorbet

Serves 4	
Per serving:	
Calories:	85.00
Protein:	0.00 g
Carbohydrates:	20.00 g
Total fat:	1.00 g
Sat. fat:	0.00 g
Cholesterol:	0.00 mg
Sodium:	0.50 mg
Fiber:	0.00 g

4 cups seeded cubed watermelon
2 tablespoons water
1 teaspoon unflavored gelatin
2 tablespoons lime juice
2 tablespoons honey

1. If you're using an ice-cream freezer, place the watermelon cubes in the freezer while you prepare the gelatin. Add the water to a microwave-safe bowl and sprinkle the gelatin over it; let stand for 2 minutes or until the gelatin softens. Microwave on high for 40 seconds; stir until the gelatin is dissolved. Pour into a blender or food processor and add half of the watermelon, the lime juice, and honey. Cover and process until smooth. Add the remaining melon and process until smooth. Pour into prepared ice-cream maker (see manufacturer's instructions); put the cover in place and plug in the machine. The mixture will take about 15 to 20 minutes to freeze.
2. If you're not using an ice-cream freezer, pour the melon mixture into ice cube trays treated with nonstick spray; freeze until firm. If your blender can make shaved ice, transfer the cubes to the blender and process. Otherwise, transfer to a chilled bowl and beat with an electric mixer until the mixture is bright pink.
3. You can put the sorbet in serving dishes and place them in the freezer until needed. If you do so, remove from the freezer about 20 minutes before you plan to serve, or at the beginning of the meal.

❋ Seasoning Popcorn
You defeat the purpose of healthful, air-popped popcorn if you drown it in butter and smother it with salt. Instead, squirt a little natural butter-flavored spray oil (like Spectrum Naturals Canola Spray Oil with Butter Flavor) over it and sprinkle on your favorite herb seasoning blend. For those times that only a salty snack will do, use Sesame Salt (page 254) instead of all salt.

Apple-Apricot Frozen Yogurt

1 large Golden Delicious apple,
peeled, cored, and diced
¼ cup Muir Glen Organic Frozen
Apple Juice Concentrate
¾ cup cold water

4 apricots, peeled (optional) and
pitted
1 large banana, peeled and sliced
¾ cup plain nonfat yogurt
1 tablespoon honey

Serves 4	
Per serving:	
Calories:	149.04
Protein:	3.38 g
Carbohydrates:	34.77 g
Total fat:	0.57 g
Sat. fat:	0.15 g
Cholesterol:	0.85 mg
Sodium:	37.28 mg
Fiber:	3.10 g

1. Add the apple, apple juice concentrate, water, apricots, and banana to a blender or food processor; process until smooth. Stir in the remaining ingredients. Add to ice-cream freezer and freeze according to manufacturer's directions.
2. If you're not using an ice-cream freezer, pour the mixture into ice cube trays treated with nonstick spray; freeze until firm. If your blender can make shaved ice, transfer the cubes to the blender and process. Otherwise, transfer to a chilled bowl and beat with an electric mixer until the mixture is whipped.

❋ Sensible Soft Drinks

Soft drinks are notoriously high in sodium. You can still have your fizzy drinks and have them sodium-free if you add ¼ cup of your favorite sodium-free frozen fruit juice concentrate to a glass and add ¾ cup of seltzer or carbonated water. (Do not use club soda because it is not sodium-free; using club soda would add about 40 milligrams of sodium to what would otherwise be a sodium-free drink.)

Fruit Mold

Serves 8	
Per serving:	
Calories:	56.71
Protein:	1.13 g
Carbohydrates:	13.73 g
Total fat:	0.11 g
Sat. fat:	0.03 g
Cholesterol:	0.00 mg
Sodium:	4.54 mg
Fiber:	0.95 g

1 envelope KNOX Unflavored
   Gelatine
¼ cup cold water
1½ cups hot water
¼ cup fresh lemon or lime juice
3 tablespoons peach or apricot
   preserves

1 tablespoon granulated sugar
1 large banana, peeled and sliced
1 cup unsweetened canned peach
   slices, drained

In a blender container, soak the gelatin in the cold water for 2 minutes. Add the hot water and blend for about 2 minutes, until the gelatin is dissolved. Add the juice, preserves, and sugar; blend until the sugar is dissolved. Stir in the banana and peach slices. Pour into a dish or mold and refrigerate until set, about 4 hours.

Triple Fruit Mold

Serves 6	
Per serving:	
Calories:	76.91
Protein:	2.16 g
Carbohydrates:	17.67 g
Total fat:	0.35 g
Sat. fat:	0.08 g
Cholesterol:	0.00 mg
Sodium:	8.91 mg
Fiber:	1.80 g

2 envelopes KNOX Unflavored
   Gelatine
½ cup frozen, unsweetened apple
   juice concentrate

3 cups unsweetened sparkling water
1 cup sliced strawberries
1 cup blueberries
2 large bananas, peeled and sliced

1. Mix together the gelatin and apple juice in a small saucepan; let stand for 1 minute. Stir the gelatin over low heat until completely dissolved, about 3 minutes. Let cool slightly.
2. Stir in the sparkling water. Refrigerate until the mixture begins to gel or is the consistency of unbeaten egg whites when stirred, about 15 minutes. (Be careful not to chill too long or it will solidify and you won't be able to add the fruit.)
3. Fold the fruit into the partially thickened gelatin mixture. Pour into a 6-cup mold. Refrigerate for 4 hours or until set.

Baked Apples

2 large apples, cored and cut in
   half
2 teaspoons lemon juice
4 teaspoons brown sugar
4 teaspoons oatmeal

Spectrum Naturals Canola Spray
   Oil with Butter Flavor
⅛ cup water

Serves 4	
Per serving:	
Calories:	100.48
Protein:	1.03 g
Carbohydrates:	24.46 g
Total fat:	0.70 g
Sat. fat:	0.12 g
Cholesterol:	0.00 mg
Sodium:	2.04 mg
Fiber:	3.42 g

1. Preheat oven to 375°. Treat an ovenproof dish with nonstick cooking spray.
2. Place the apples cut-side up in the prepared dish. Brush 1 teaspoon of the lemon juice over each apple. In a small bowl, mix together the brown sugar and oatmeal; evenly divide over the apples. Mist the top of the apples with the spray oil. Add the water to the bottom of the baking dish. Bake for 35 minutes or until the apples are fork tender. Serve hot or cold.

❀ Sugar Subsitute

Whey Low powder (see Appendix B) is an all-natural, low-glycemic sugar substitute (with only 25 percent of the calories of sugar) that can be used measure-for-measure the same as sugar, plus it's safe to use in baking.

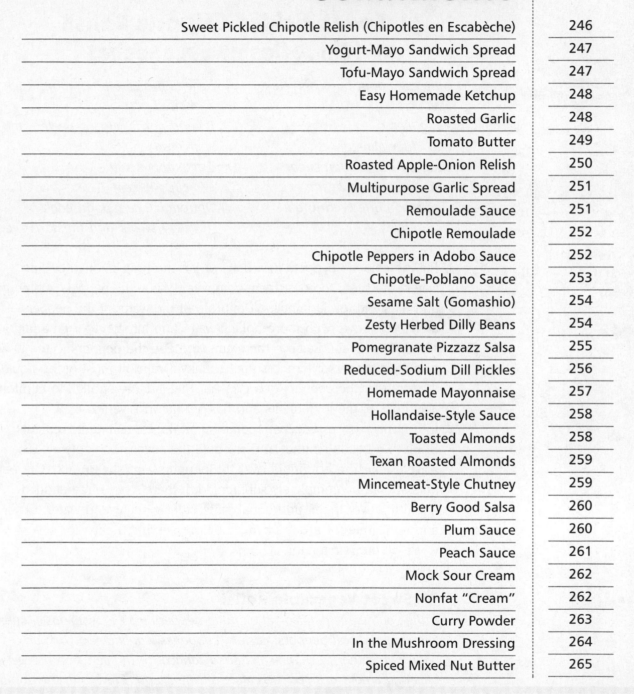

CHAPTER 14 ❦
Condiments

Sweet Pickled Chipotle Relish
(Chipotles en Escabèche)

Serves 48	
Per serving:	
Calories:	13.12
Protein:	0.13 g
Carbohydrates:	3.36 g
Total fat:	0.04 g
Sat. fat:	0.01 g
Cholesterol:	0.00 mg
Sodium:	98.55 mg
Fiber:	0.23 g

4 ounces (about 50) chipotle peppers
Boiling water
1 cup cider vinegar
½ packed cup brown sugar
½ teaspoon dried thyme
½ teaspoon dried marjoram
3 bay leaves
1 medium-size white onion, finely minced
1 head garlic, cloves peeled and minced
2 teaspoons salt
1¼ cups water
Optional: 1 teaspoon each of celery seeds and mustard seeds

1. Put the chipotle peppers in a bowl or jar and pour enough boiling water over them to cover them completely. Keep the peppers submerged and let stand for 10 minutes. Drain off all the water. If the peppers aren't soft, cover with more boiling water and let stand for an additional 10 minutes. Drain. Remove the stems and add the peppers to the bowl of a food processor; process until chunky. Drain off most of the liquid, then transfer the peppers to a glass jar that is large enough to comfortably hold all the ingredients and has a noncorrosive lid.

2. In a noncorrosive saucepan, combine all the remaining ingredients. Bring to a gentle simmer and stir until the sugar is completely dissolved. Pour the hot liquid over the peppers and stir to mix. The peppers should be completely submerged; if there's not quite enough liquid to cover them, add equal parts cider vinegar and water. Cover and refrigerate for a day or more before serving. Keeps for several weeks in the refrigerator.

❀ Sweet Vegetable Relish
If the southwestern flavor of chipotle peppers isn't to your taste, substitute chopped bell peppers, carrots, cabbages, cauliflower, or your choices of other fresh, no-salt-added canned, or thawed frozen vegetables and create a sweet vegetable relish instead. Even with the amount of salt used in this recipe, you'll end up with a relish that only has about two-thirds the sodium of most commercial versions.

Yogurt-Mayo Sandwich Spread

¼ cup drained nonfat yogurt

¼ cup Hellmann's or Best Foods Real Mayonnaise

1. Measure the yogurt into a paper coffee filter. Wrap the filter up and around the yogurt and twist to secure. Place the filter in a strainer set to drain over a cup or bowl. Refrigerate for at least 1 hour. (While this step isn't necessary, it does help make for a creamier, thicker spread.)
2. In a small bowl, combine the drained yogurt with the mayonnaise. Use as you would mayonnaise. Store in the refrigerator in a covered container until the expiration date on the yogurt.

Serves 8	
Per serving:	
Calories:	53.27
Protein:	0.48 g
Carbohydrates:	0.73 g
Total fat:	5.47 g
Sat. fat:	0.60 g
Cholesterol:	4.20 mg
Sodium:	44.51 mg
Fiber:	0.00 g

Tofu-Mayo Sandwich Spread

2 ounces firm silken tofu

¼ cup Hellmann's or Best Foods Real Mayonnaise

In a small bowl, combine the silken tofu with the mayonnaise. Use as you would mayonnaise. This sandwich spread is best when made the night before to allow time for the flavors to meld. Store in the refrigerator in a covered container until the expiration date on the tofu.

Serves 8	
Per serving:	
Calories:	53.69
Protein:	0.56 g
Carbohydrates:	0.36 g
Total fat:	5.65 g
Sat. fat:	0.62 g
Cholesterol:	4.06 mg
Sodium:	41.60 mg
Fiber:	0.01 g

Easy Homemade Ketchup

Serves 32	
Per serving:	
Calories:	17.76
Protein:	0.12 g
Carbohydrates:	4.43 g
Total fat:	0.01 g
Sat. fat:	0.00 g
Cholesterol:	0.00 mg
Sodium:	24.74 mg
Fiber:	0.24 g

*1 (15-ounce) can Muir Glen Organic
   No Salt Added Tomato Sauce*
2 teaspoons water
½ teaspoon onion powder
½ cup granulated sugar
⅓ cup cider vinegar
¼ teaspoon sea salt
¼ teaspoon ground cinnamon
⅛ teaspoon ground cloves
Pinch ground allspice
Pinch nutmeg
Pinch freshly ground pepper
⅔ teaspoon sweet paprika

1. Add all the ingredients *except* the paprika to a nonstick saucepan. Simmer over low heat for 15 to 30 minutes, until the mixture reduces to desired consistency.
2. Remove from heat and stir in the paprika. Allow the mixture to cool, then put it in a covered container (such as a recycled ketchup bottle). Store in the refrigerator until needed.

Roasted Garlic

Servings vary	
Per serving (1 clove of garlic):	
Calories:	4.47
Protein:	0.19 g
Carbohydrates:	0.99 g
Total fat:	2.34 g
Sat. fat:	0.00 g
Cholesterol:	0.00 mg
Sodium:	0.51 mg
Fiber:	0.06 g

1 or more garlic heads

1. Preheat oven to 350°.
2. Lightly spray a small baking dish with nonstick spray. Slice off ½" from the top of each garlic head and rub off any loose skins, being careful not to separate the cloves. Place the garlic in baking dish, cut-side up; if roasting more than 1 head of garlic, arrange them in the dish so that they don't touch. Cover and bake until the garlic cloves are very tender when pierced, about 30 to 45 minutes.
3. To serve, squeeze cloves from their skins directly onto bread and use a knife to spread.

Tomato Butter

½ teaspoon saffron threads
¼ cup Mushroom Broth (page 164)
4 cups fresh tomatoes, peeled,
seeded, and diced
½ pound unsalted butter, at room
temperature

2 tablespoons white wine vinegar
½ teaspoon salt
Pinch freshly ground black pepper

Serves 20	
Per serving:	
Calories:	95.96
Protein:	0.66 g
Carbohydrates:	3.27 g
Total fat:	8.76 g
Sat. fat:	5.73 g
Cholesterol:	24.00 mg
Sodium:	69.26 mg
Fiber:	0.30 g

1. Combine the saffron and broth in a small bowl; let stand for 15 minutes.
2. Bring a large, deep nonstick sauté pan to temperature over medium heat. Add the tomatoes and broth to the pan; bring to a boil, then lower heat. Simmer the tomatoes, stirring frequently, for 40 to 45 minutes or until the mixture is very thick and reduced in volume to less than 1 cup.
3. Add the butter several tablespoons at a time, whisking after each addition until it has been incorporated into the tomatoes. Add the vinegar, salt, and pepper. Can be stored in the refrigerator for several days or frozen for 3 months.

❀ Tomato Butter Tips
If you prefer not to take the time to peel and seed the tomatoes before cooking them, you can coarse-chop them instead. Prepare the recipe as directed; however, once it's been seasoned, force the mixture through a fine-meshed sieve using the back of a spoon to remove the seeds and skins.

Roasted Apple-Onion Relish

Serves 8	
Per serving:	
Calories:	21.38
Protein:	0.18 g
Carbohydrates:	5.55 g
Total fat:	0.05 g
Sat. fat:	0.01 g
Cholesterol:	0.00 mg
Sodium:	1.08 mg
Fiber:	0.63 g

Spectrum Naturals Canola Spray
   Oil with Butter Flavor
1 small sweet onion, minced
1 tart cooking apple, peeled,
   cored, and chopped
1 cup unsweetened, no-salt-added
   applesauce
1 tablespoon apple cider vinegar

1 teaspoon Muir Glen Organic frozen
   Apple Juice Concentrate or honey
1 tablespoon lemon juice
1/8 teaspoon dried thyme
1/8 teaspoon freshly ground black
   pepper
Pinch dried orange granules,
   crushed

1. Preheat oven to 400°. Treat a baking tray or rectangular ovenproof casserole dish with the spray oil.
2. Mix together the chopped apple and minced onion; add to the prepared tray or dish and spread out in a single layer. Lightly spray with the spray oil. Bake for 10 minutes. Stir the mixture. Bake for 5 to 10 minutes, until tender and lightly browned.
3. Bring a small nonstick saucepan to temperature over low heat. Add the roasted apple-onion mixture and all of the remaining ingredients; simmer for 15 to 20 minutes, stirring frequently, until the mixture is reduced by half and light to medium brown in color. Note: Increase the stirring frequency halfway through and until the end of the cooking time, as the relish can easily burn once it's reduced.

❈ Storing Roasted Garlic

Roasted garlic heads can be kept in the refrigerator for 2 or 3 days. To keep them longer, squeeze the roasted garlic into a container and cover completely with olive oil. Cover tightly and refrigerate. This creates a garlic-infused olive oil that can be used in salads or sautés.

Multipurpose Garlic Spread

1 ounce Parmesan cheese, cubed
4 cloves roasted garlic (page 248)
1 teaspoon Grey Poupon Dijon
   mustard
1 teaspoon dry white wine

½ teaspoon Lea & Perrin
   Worcestershire sauce
Pinch freshly ground black pepper
½ cup silken firm tofu
1 tablespoon extra-virgin olive oil

Serves 8	
Per 1-tablespoon serving:	
Calories:	35.64
Protein:	2.71 g
Carbohydrates:	1.15 g
Total fat:	2.27 g
Sat. fat:	0.84 g
Cholesterol:	2.80 mg
Sodium:	86.47 mg
Fiber:	0.09 g

1. Put the cheese cubes into a blender container and chop them on the lowest speed until the cheese settles into the bottom; gradually increase the speed until the cheese is grated.
2. Add the garlic, mustard, wine, Worcestershire sauce, pepper, and tofu to the blender; blend until smooth.
3. While the blender is running, drizzle in the olive oil and continue to process until mixed with the other spread ingredients.

Remoulade Sauce

½ cup Hellmann's or Best Foods
   Real Mayonnaise
½ cup plain nonfat yogurt
1 tablespoon lemon juice
1 tablespoon Cascadian Farm Dill
   Relish
1 teaspoon capers, rinsed and
   crushed

1 tablespoon freeze-dried shallot
1 teaspoon freeze-dried chives
½ teaspoon dried parsley
¼ teaspoon freshly ground white
   or black pepper

Serves 18	
Per serving:	
Calories:	29.40
Protein:	0.43 g
Carbohydrates:	2.16 g
Total fat:	2.19 g
Sat. fat:	0.33 g
Cholesterol:	1.82 mg
Sodium:	64.34 mg
Fiber:	0.01 g

In a bowl, combine all the ingredients until well blended. Refrigerate until needed. Can be safely stored in the refrigerator until the expiration date on the yogurt.

Chipotle Remoulade

Serves 32	
Per serving:	
Calories:	13.00
Protein:	0.30 g
Carbohydrates:	1.73 g
Total fat:	0.64 g
Sat. fat:	0.10 g
Cholesterol:	0.55 mg
Sodium:	34.58 mg
Fiber:	0.09 g

1 cup Chipotle Peppers in Adobo Sauce
2 teaspoons lime juice
¼ cup Hellmann's or Best Foods Real Mayonnaise
½ cup plain nonfat yogurt
¼ cup minced fresh cilantro
⅛ teaspoon freshly ground black pepper

Put the Chipotle Peppers in Adobo Sauce and lime juice in a blender or food processor; process until smooth. Transfer to a bowl and mix together with the remaining ingredients. Refrigerate until needed. Can be safely stored in the refrigerator until the expiration date on the yogurt.

Chipotle Peppers in Adobo Sauce

Serves 8	
Per serving:	
Calories:	15.06
Protein:	0.31 g
Carbohydrates:	3.94 g
Total fat:	0.07 g
Sat. fat:	0.01 g
Cholesterol:	0.00 mg
Sodium:	75.05 mg
Fiber:	0.35 g

7 medium-sized dried chipotle chilies
⅓ cup chopped white or yellow onion
5 tablespoons apple cider vinegar
2 cloves garlic, sliced
4 tablespoons low-sodium ketchup
¼ teaspoon salt
3 cups boiling water

1. Remove the stems and seeds from the chilies, and slit the chilies lengthwise. Roast in a heavy skillet over medium-high heat, turning them occasionally; heat until puffed and just beginning to get brown, about 10 seconds each. (Do not burn the peppers or the resulting sauce will be bitter.)
2. Combine all of the ingredients in a nonreactive pan and pour the boiling water over them. Cover and cook over very low heat for 1 to 1½ hours, until the chilies are very soft and the liquid has been reduced to 1 cup. Freeze leftovers, or they can be kept for several weeks in the refrigerator in an airtight container.

Chipotle-Poblano Sauce

6 chipotle peppers
1 poblano pepper
½ cup boiling water
½ teaspoon cumin seed
½ teaspoon dried Mexican oregano

1 tablespoon dried minced onion
1 teaspoon onion powder
2 teaspoons roasted garlic powder
1 tablespoon olive oil
Pinch salt

Serves 10	
Per serving:	
Calories:	17.49
Protein:	0.20 g
Carbohydrates:	1.26 g
Total fat:	1.38 g
Sat. fat:	0.19 g
Cholesterol:	0.00 mg
Sodium:	29.78 mg
Fiber:	0.22 g

1. Remove the stems and seeds from the peppers, and slit the peppers lengthwise. Roast in a heavy skillet over medium-high heat, turning them occasionally; heat until puffed and just beginning to get brown, about 10 seconds each. (Do not burn the peppers or the resulting sauce will be bitter.) As they're done, put the peppers in a bowl.
2. Pour the boiling water over the peppers; let soak for 15 minutes. (If you wish to peel the peppers, remove them from the water with a slotted spoon and do so before completing step 4.)
3. Dry-roast the cumin and oregano in the skillet until fragrant, being careful that the oregano doesn't burn.
4. Add all the ingredients to the bowl of a food processor or blender container. Process until mixed, yet still chunky. Leftovers can be stored for several days in the refrigerator.

❁ Crispy Alternative to Pickles

Try a ¼-cup serving of the Zesty Herbed Dilly Bean recipe (page 254) on a hamburger instead of dill pickles and you'll have that traditional All-American flavor at a fraction of the sodium content. Green beans are blanched before frozen, so using a package of frozen beans saves you that step and they are crisper than using no-salt-added canned green beans.

Sesame Salt (Gomashio)

Serves 40	
Per serving:	
Calories:	3.40
Protein:	0.10 g
Carbohydrates:	0.16 g
Total fat:	0.29 g
Sat. fat:	0.04 g
Cholesterol:	0.00 mg
Sodium:	59.18 mg
Fiber:	0.10 g

3 tablespoons sesame seeds   *1 teaspoon sea salt*

1. Toast the sesame seeds in a heavy skillet over medium heat until they're light brown and aromatic. (The seeds may start to "pop" at this point.) Stir frequently to prevent the seeds from burning. Set aside to cool.
2. Add the salt to the toasted sesame seeds and mix well. Grind with a mortar and pestle until the seeds crack open; the mixture will be a coarse grind. (Alternatively, you can put the mixture in a bowl and "grind" it with the back of a spoon, or, grind it in a spice grinder or food processor and pulse the mixture a few times.) Regardless of the method you use, do not overprocess it. Like peanuts, sesame seeds have natural oils that will turn it into a paste if you process it too much, and you'll end up with nut butter.

Zesty Herbed Dilly Beans

Serves 16	
Per serving:	
Calories:	13.19
Protein:	0.75 g
Carbohydrates:	2.98 g
Total fat:	0.05 g
Sat. fat:	0.00 g
Cholesterol:	0.00 mg
Sodium:	73.04 mg
Fiber:	0.75 g

1 (16-ounce) package Cascadian Farms Organic frozen Green Beans, thawed
¾ cup apple cider vinegar
¾ cup water
¼ teaspoon cayenne pepper or dried red pepper flakes

2 cloves garlic, minced
2 teaspoons dill seeds
1 teaspoon dried dill weed
½ teaspoon salt

1. Put the thawed green beans in a glass jar or other covered container large enough to hold the beans and vinegar mixture.
2. In a medium nonreactive saucepan over high heat, bring the vinegar and water to a boil. Stir in the cayenne pepper (or pepper flakes), garlic, dill seeds and weed, and salt. Pour the vinegar mixture over the green beans. Allow to cool to room temperature.
3. Cover and refrigerate for 24 hours before serving.

Pomegranate Pizzazz Salsa

1 large banana, peeled and chopped
2 limes, zested and juiced
1 teaspoon pomegranate molasses
1 clove garlic, minced
1 jalapeño, seeded and minced
2 teaspoons Citrus Pepper (page 278)
¼ teaspoon mustard powder or Dijon mustard
Pinch (or to taste) dried red pepper flakes

Optional: 1 tablespoon water
1 large red or sweet onion, chopped
2 avocadoes, pitted, peeled, and diced
¼ cup chopped fresh cilantro
2 large tomatoes, peeled, seeded, and chopped
2 large peaches, peeled, pitted, and chopped
Optional: Freshly ground pepper

Serves 16	
Per serving:	
Calories:	68.58
Protein:	1.11 g
Carbohydrates:	9.08 g
Total fat:	4.02 g
Sat. fat:	0.65 g
Cholesterol:	0.00 mg
Sodium:	5.25 mg
Fiber:	2.54 g

Add the banana, lime zest and juice, pomegranate molasses, garlic, jalapeño, Citrus Pepper, mustard powder (or Dijon), and red pepper flakes to a blender or food processor; process until smooth. If the resulting banana-lime mixture is thicker than you prefer, add the optional water at this time and pulse to combine. Add the onion, avocadoes, cilantro, tomatoes, and peaches to a bowl; stir to mix. Pour the banana-lime mixture over the ingredients in the bowl and toss gently. Serve immediately. (If preparing in advance, add the avocado at the last minute.)

❋ Substitution Suggestions

Pomegranate Pizzazz Salsa is another versatile recipe; you can substitute mango for the peaches and/or Cascadian Farm Frozen Organic Raspberry or Orange Juice Concentrate for the pomegranate concentrate or molasses. If you're making salsa for a huge crowd, you can go crazy and even throw in some cooked sweet corn and chopped red and green bell pepper, too.

Reduced-Sodium Dill Pickles

Serves 16	
Per serving:	
Calories:	22.51
Protein:	1.00 g
Carbohydrates:	5.28 g
Total fat:	0.17 g
Sat. fat:	0.02 g
Cholesterol:	0.00 mg
Sodium:	146.87 mg
Fiber:	1.07 g

1½ cups white wine vinegar
½ cup water
2 teaspoons honey
¼ teaspoon red pepper flakes
1 teaspoon whole white peppercorns
1 teaspoon coriander seeds

1 teaspoon mustard seeds
½ teaspoon fennel seeds
½ teaspoon toasted cumin seeds
1 tablespoon kosher salt
2 teaspoons dried dill weed
1 teaspoon dried cilantro
2 large cucumbers

1. Combine the vinegar, water, honey, pepper flakes, peppercorns, coriander seeds, mustard seeds, fennel seeds, cumin seeds, and salt in a medium-size nonreactive saucepan over high heat; bring to a boil. Remove from heat and set aside to let cool to room temperature. Add the dill and cilantro.
2. Wash the cucumbers, cut them in half horizontally, and then quarter them lengthwise. (Removing the seeds or peeling from the cucumbers is optional.) Place the cucumber sections in a covered container and pour the cooled vinegar mixture over them. Refrigerate, covered, for 24 hours. Use within 1 week.

❊ Have Your Dill

Be creative with either the dilly beans or dill pickle recipe. Convert the dilly bean recipe to a dilled 3-bean salad by adding some cooked white and pinto beans and a little chopped celery. Or, substitute any canned no-salt-added vegetable for the cucumbers in the latter recipe. Chopped fresh bell pepper is good in either recipe, as is sliced or chopped onion. If the dilly beans or dill pickles simply aren't salty enough for your taste, try adding some lemon juice to them before adding any additional salt. If either recipe is too tart for your taste, increase the amount of water in the recipe.

Homemade Mayonnaise

¾ cup cold water
1 tablespoon cornstarch
2 large egg yolks
1 tablespoon (or more, to taste)
  lemon juice
Optional: Choice of freshly ground
  pepper, to taste

1 teaspoon (or more, to taste)
  Grey Poupon Dijon Mustard
1 cup canola oil
Optional: Sea salt (or other easy-
  to-dissolve salt; do not use
  kosher salt)

Serves 32	
Per serving:	
Calories:	65.16
Protein:	0.18 g
Carbohydrates:	0.30 g
Total fat:	7.13 g
Sat. fat:	0.58 g
Cholesterol:	13.29 mg
Sodium:	4.22 mg
Fiber:	0.00 g

1. In a small nonstick saucepan, whisk together the water and cornstarch; bring to a boil over medium-high heat. While the cornstarch-water mixture comes to temperature, add the egg yolks and lemon juice to a small bowl and whisk until they're lighter in color and foamy. Once the cornstarch begins to gel, slowly pour the egg mixture into the saucepan, whisking constantly as you do. Add the pepper, if using. Return the mixture in the pan to a boil and whisk until it just begins to thicken. Set aside, or pour into a bowl, and let cool completely.

2. Once the mixture is cool, whisk in the mustard by hand or use a mixer set on medium speed. With the mixer running, or whisking constantly, slowly add the oil. Taste the mayonnaise and whisk in additional lemon juice, mustard, or up to ¼ teaspoon salt, if desired. Strain into a small bowl, cover, and refrigerate for a minimum of 2 hours. (At this point the mayonnaise will seem somewhat runny or fluid; however, it will thicken once refrigerated.)

3. Upon removal from the refrigerator, it may be necessary to whisk the mixture again; if there has been any separation, whisking it while adding 1 teaspoon of water at a time will cause the mayonnaise to emulsify once more. Keep refrigerated; can be safely stored for several days.

Hollandaise-Style Sauce

Serves 8	
Per serving:	
Calories:	67.32
Protein:	0.19 g
Carbohydrates:	0.90 g
Total fat:	7.13 g
Sat. fat:	0.58 g
Cholesterol:	13.30 mg
Sodium:	4.24 mg
Fiber:	0.01 g

½ cup Homemade Mayonnaise (page 257)
1 tablespoon fresh lemon juice
1–2 tablespoons Mr. Spice Honey Mustard Sauce
Pinch dried red pepper flakes, crushed
Freshly ground black pepper, to taste

Add all the ingredients to a small serving bowl and whisk to combine. Refrigerate leftovers; can be safely kept (covered) in the refrigerator for several days.

Toasted Almonds

Serves 24	
Per serving:	
Calories:	17.16
Protein:	0.64 g
Carbohydrates:	0.55 g
Total fat:	1.52 g
Sat. fat:	0.12 g
Cholesterol:	0.00 mg
Sodium:	0.03 mg
Fiber:	0.34 g

½ cup ground raw almonds

Add the raw almonds to a nonstick skillet over low heat. Toast until golden, shaking the pan or stirring the nuts frequently so that they toast evenly. When the nuts reach a light brown color, remove from the heat and pour into a bowl. Allow to cool completely, then store in an airtight container kept in a cool, dry place.

Texan Roasted Almonds

Serves 16	
Per serving:	
Calories:	57.44
Protein:	2.00 g
Carbohydrates:	1.92 g
Total fat:	5.07 g
Sat. fat:	0.65 g
Cholesterol:	1.29 mg
Sodium:	4.67 mg
Fiber:	0.96 g

2 teaspoons unsalted butter
½ teaspoon Lea & Perrins
Worcestershire sauce
½ teaspoon Texas Seasoning
(page 275)
1 cup slivered almonds

1. Preheat oven to 350°.
2. In a microwave-safe bowl, mix together the butter, Worcestershire sauce, and Texas Seasoning; microwave on high for 30 seconds or until the butter is melted; stir well.
3. Spread the almonds on a shallow baking sheet treated with nonstick spray. Bake for 12 to 15 minutes or until light gold, stirring occasionally. Pour the seasoned butter over the almonds, and stir to mix. Return to the oven and bake for 5 minutes. Cool, then store in airtight containers in a cool place.

Mincemeat-Style Chutney

Serves 48	
Per serving:	
Calories:	14.04
Protein:	0.14 g
Carbohydrates:	3.38 g
Total fat:	0.05 g
Sat. fat:	0.01 g
Cholesterol:	0.00 mg
Sodium:	0.34 mg
Fiber:	0.38 g

1 cup diced sweet onion
1 cup peeled and diced Granny
Smith apples
1 cup peeled and diced bananas
1 cup peeled and diced peaches
¼ cup raisins
¼ cup dried cranberries
¼ cup dry white wine
¼ cup apple cider vinegar
1 teaspoon brown sugar
½ teaspoon cinnamon
½ teaspoon Pumpkin Pie Spice
(page 275)
⅛ teaspoon ground black pepper
⅛ teaspoon dried lemon granules,
crushed

In a large saucepan, combine all the ingredients and cook over low heat for about 1 hour, stirring occasionally. Let cool completely. Can be kept for 1 week in the refrigerator or in the freezer for 3 months.

Berry Good Salsa

Serves 16	
Per serving:	
Calories:	23.56
Protein:	0.42 g
Carbohydrates:	5.94 g
Total fat:	0.10 g
Sat. fat:	0.02 g
Cholesterol:	0.00 mg
Sodium:	4.68 mg
Fiber:	1.02 g

1 cup blackberries
½ cantaloupe, diced
1 jalapeño or banana pepper, diced
1 small red or green bell pepper, diced
1 medium-size red onion, diced
1 tablespoon lemon juice
⅛ teaspoon freshly ground black pepper

Pinch mustard powder
⅛ teaspoon dried lemon granules, crushed
½ teaspoon dried cilantro or parsley
½ teaspoon Texas Seasoning (page 275)

Place all the ingredients in a food processor and process until well mixed. Do not overprocess—the salsa should remain somewhat chunky.

Plum Sauce

Serves 20	
Per serving:	
Calories:	28.74
Protein:	0.01 g
Carbohydrates:	7.51 g
Total fat:	0.00 g
Sat. fat:	0.00 g
Cholesterol:	0.00 mg
Sodium:	0.03 mg
Fiber:	0.02 g

1 cup Smucker's Plum Jam
½ teaspoon dried lemon granules, crushed
1 tablespoon lemon juice
1 tablespoon rice wine or white wine vinegar
½ teaspoon ground dried ginger

½ teaspoon crushed anise seeds
¼ teaspoon dry mustard
¼ teaspoon ground cinnamon
⅛ teaspoon ground cloves
⅛ teaspoon Mr. Spice Tangy Bang! Hot Sauce

Heat the plum jam in a small saucepan over medium heat until melted. Stir in the remaining ingredients. Bring the mixture to a boil, lower the heat, and simmer for 1 minute, stirring constantly.

Peach Sauce

2 teaspoons olive oil

1 tablespoon chopped shallot

1 teaspoon grated fresh ginger

⅛ teaspoon dried lemon granules, crushed

½ teaspoon Pumpkin Pie Spice (page 275)

Pinch mustard powder

⅓ cup dry white wine

1 small peach, peeled and diced

1 tablespoon Cascadian Farm Organic Frozen Unsweetened Orange Juice Concentrate

1 teaspoon Bragg Liquid Aminos

½ teaspoon cornstarch

Serves 4	
Per serving:	
Calories:	53.57
Protein:	0.56 g
Carbohydrates:	4.97 g
Total fat:	2.29 g
Sat. fat:	0.31 g
Cholesterol:	0.00 mg
Sodium:	56.58 mg
Fiber:	0.45 g

1. Heat the olive oil in a nonstick saucepan over medium heat; sauté the shallot and ginger until soft. Add the lemon granules, Pumpkin Pie Spice, mustard powder, and wine; simmer until reduced by half. Add the diced peach, orange juice concentrate, and Bragg Liquid Aminos and bring to a simmer, stirring occasionally.

2. In a separate container, mix the cornstarch with 1 tablespoon of the sauce; stir to create a slurry, mixing well to remove any lumps. Add the slurry to the sauce and simmer until the mixture thickens. Transfer the mixture to a blender or food processor container and process until smooth.

❋ A Fat Is Still Fattening

Keep in mind that even when you use a healthier, nonhydrogenated oil shortening like Spectrum Naturals Organic All-Vegetable Shortening, it's still a fat. Each tablespoon of that shortening has 110 calories (13 grams of fat; 6 grams of saturated fat). You can sometimes substitute plain nonfat yogurt or applesauce for some of or all of the fat called for in a recipe. (Unfortunately, finding out which can be substituted takes some experimentation. The "all" substitution works best in moist banana or zucchini bread recipes.)

Serves 6	
Per serving:	
Calories:	11.72
Protein:	1.36 g
Carbohydrates:	0.62 g
Total fat:	0.40 g
Sat. fat:	0.26 g
Cholesterol:	1.41 mg
Sodium:	39.08 mg
Fiber:	0.00 g

Mock Sour Cream

⅛ *cup plain nonfat yogurt*   ½ *teaspoon vinegar*
¼ *cup cottage cheese*

Put all the ingredients in a blender or food processor; process until smooth.

❁ Vinegar Options

The type of vinegar used in the Mock Sour Cream recipe will affect the "tang" of the sour cream taste. Apple cider vinegar, for example, has a stronger taste; white wine or champagne vinegar tends to be milder.

Serves 4	
Per serving:	
Calories:	36.65
Protein:	3.58 g
Carbohydrates:	5.19 g
Total fat:	0.14 g
Sat. fat:	0.09 g
Cholesterol:	1.99 mg
Sodium:	55.18 mg
Fiber:	0.00 g

Nonfat "Cream"

1 cup skim milk   ¼ *cup nonfat dry milk*

Add the milk and nonfat dry milk to a blender or food processor; process until mixed.

Curry Powder

1 tablespoon coriander seeds
½ tablespoon cumin seeds
½ teaspoon fennel seeds
¼ teaspoon whole cloves or
⅛ teaspoon ground cloves
¼ teaspoon mustard seeds
½ tablespoon cardamom seeds

½ tablespoon whole black peppercorns
½ teaspoon dried red pepper flakes, or crushed red peppers
½ tablespoon turmeric
⅛ teaspoon ground ginger
⅛ teaspoon ground cinnamon

Yields about ¼ cup	
Per serving:	
Calories:	1.23
Protein:	0.05 g
Carbohydrates:	0.21 g
Total fat:	0.06 g
Sat. fat:	0.01 g
Cholesterol:	0.00 mg
Sodium:	0.23 mg
Fiber:	0.10 g

1. Toast the coriander seeds, cumin seeds, fennel seeds, cloves, mustard seeds, cardamom seeds, peppercorns, and red pepper flakes in a small, dry skillet over medium-low heat. Stir the spices often to prevent them from burning. Toast for a couple of minutes, or until the spices smell fragrant.

2. Add the toasted spices to a clean coffee grinder (see Appendix B) and grind into a fine powder. Add the turmeric, ginger, and cinnamon, and pulse the grinder a few times to combine them with the other spices. Use the spice blend immediately, or, if stored in a sealed glass jar, it can be kept in a cool, dry place for 1 month or indefinitely in the freezer.

❀ Currying a Flavor

A dry-toasted curry powder blend lets you eliminate some of the butter or oil called for in a recipe because the fat isn't needed to sauté the powder, although the fat can be left in the recipe for the extra flavor it imparts—or if it's needed to make a roux—if leaving it is within the fat requirements of your diet.

In the Mushroom Dressing

Serves 12	
Per serving:	
Calories:	39.28
Protein:	2.86 g
Carbohydrates:	5.02 g
Total fat:	1.17 g
Sat. fat:	0.31 g
Cholesterol:	35.48 mg
Sodium:	37.27 mg
Fiber:	0.79 g

24 large button mushrooms, cleaned, stems removed and chopped
Spectrum Naturals Extra-Virgin Olive Spray Oil with Garlic Flavor
¼ teaspoon Minor's Low Sodium Chicken Base
¼ cup water
1 large sweet onion, chopped
⅛ teaspoon freshly ground black pepper
⅛ teaspoon mustard powder
½–1 teaspoon Stuffing Blend (page 275)
1 cup bread crumbs
2 large eggs, beaten

1. Preheat oven to 400°.
2. Lightly mist the tops and bottoms of the mushroom caps with the spray oil. Arrange in an ovenproof casserole dish or roasting pan, stem-side up.
3. Put the base and water in a microwave-safe bowl; microwave on high for 30 seconds. Stir to mix the base with the water. Add the chopped mushroom stems and onion; cover and microwave on high for 3 to 5 minutes, until the onion is tender and transparent. Set aside to cool.
4. Stir the pepper, mustard powder, Stuffing Blend, bread crumbs, and eggs into the onion-broth mixture. Evenly divide the mixture between the mushroom caps, spooning approximately 2 teaspoons of the bread crumb mixture into each cap. Lightly mist the stuffed mushroom caps with the spray oil. Bake for 20 to 25 minutes or until the mushrooms are tender when pierced with a fork.

❀ Sage Advice
While dried sage is a staple in most stuffing blends, its flavor is too strong for some tastes. If you prefer, you can omit the dried sage in the Stuffing Blend and increase the marjoram to 2 tablespoons and add 1 tablespoon of dried thyme.

Spiced Mixed Nut Butter

⅛ cup sesame seeds
⅛ cup ground almonds
⅛ cup sunflower seeds
½ tablespoon honey
¼ teaspoon cinnamon

⅛ teaspoon Pumpkin Pie Spice
(page 275)
Pinch unsweetened cocoa powder
Pinch dried lemon granules,
crushed

Serves 8	
Per serving:	
Calories:	38.66
Protein:	1.24 g
Carbohydrates:	2.44 g
Total fat:	2.99 g
Sat. fat:	0.33 g
Cholesterol:	0.00 mg
Sodium:	0.42 mg
Fiber:	0.76 g

1. Bring a large, deep nonstick sauté pan to temperature over medium heat. Add the sesame seeds, ground almonds, and sunflower seeds; toast for 5 to 7 minutes or until lightly browned, stirring frequently to prevent burning. Immediately transfer the nuts to a bowl and let cool.
2. Combine the cooled, toasted nuts along with the remaining ingredients in a blender or food processor; process until the desired consistency is reached, scraping down the sides of the bowl as necessary. (Note: A mini food processor works best for a recipe this size.)

❁ Nut Butter Goodness
Serve Spiced Mixed Nut Butter with toast points, crackers, or celery sticks. Refrigerate any leftovers.

CHAPTER 15
Lunchbox Favorites

Easy Tomato Basil Soup

Serves 1	
Per serving:	
Calories:	31.15
Protein:	1.54 g
Carbohydrates:	5.50 g
Total fat:	0.91 g
Sat. fat:	0.33 g
Cholesterol:	0.90 mg
Sodium:	146.11 mg
Fiber:	0.68 g

1 cup boiling water
¾ teaspoon Minor's Low Sodium Chicken Base
1 teaspoon freeze-dried basil
⅛ teaspoon freshly ground black pepper

Pinch dried red pepper flakes
1 tablespoon freeze-dried shallot
4 wedges of Oven-Dried Seasoned Tomatoes (page 194), diced

1. Prepare a 10-ounce, wide-mouth thermos bottle by filling it with hot water.
2. Drain the hot water from the thermos and discard. Stir the Minor's base into the boiling water. Add the remaining ingredients and mix well. Pour the soup into the thermos and seal the lid. At lunch, either stir the soup or shake the thermos a few times to combine the ingredients.

Islands Cauliflower Soup

Serves 1	
Per serving:	
Calories:	65.30
Protein:	4.88 g
Carbohydrates:	11.31 g
Total fat:	1.49 g
Sat. fat:	0.36 g
Cholesterol:	0.60 mg
Sodium:	127.88 mg
Fiber:	6.12 g

½ cup boiling water
½ teaspoon Minor's Low Sodium Chicken Base
½ teaspoon Caribbean Spice Blend (page 275)
⅛ teaspoon freshly ground white or black pepper

1 cup diced (unseasoned) steamed cauliflower
1 tablespoon freeze-dried green onion

1. Prepare a 10-ounce, wide-mouth thermos by filling it with hot water.
2. Drain the hot water from the thermos and discard. Stir the Minor's base into the boiling water. Add the remaining ingredients and mix well. Pour the soup into the thermos and seal the lid. At lunch, either stir the soup or shake the thermos a few times to combine the ingredients.

Broccoli and Roasted Potato Soup

Serves 1	
Per serving:	
Calories:	197.23
Protein:	6.36 g
Carbohydrates:	42.92 g
Total fat:	1.17 g
Sat. fat:	0.32 g
Cholesterol:	0.60 mg
Sodium:	125.57 mg
Fiber:	5.85 g

3 potato wedges from Oven-Fried Potato Wedges (page 177), chopped
½ cup chopped (unseasoned) steamed broccoli florets
½ cup boiling water
½ teaspoon Minor's Low Sodium Chicken Base
Optional: Country Table Spice Blend (page 275), to taste

1. Prepare a 10-ounce, wide-mouth thermos by filling it with hot water.
2. Add the potatoes and broccoli to a microwave-safe bowl; cover and microwave on high until heated through. Drain the hot water from the thermos and discard. Put the heated potatoes and broccoli in the thermos.
3. Stir the Minor's base into the boiling water; pour over the ingredients in the thermos, stir, and season to taste with the spice blend, if desired. Seal the lid. At lunch, either stir the soup or shake the thermos a few times to combine the ingredients.

Lunchbox Beef Stew

Serves 1	
Per serving:	
Calories:	252.11
Protein:	14.23 g
Carbohydrates:	43.83 g
Total fat:	2.62 g
Sat. fat:	0.91 g
Cholesterol:	25.95 mg
Sodium:	163.48 mg
Fiber:	5.64 g

1 ounce Easy Slow-Cooked "Roast" Beef (page 145), chopped
1 medium-size steamed potato, diced
½ cup unseasoned steamed carrots
¾ cup boiling water
¼ teaspoon Minor's Low Sodium Beef Base
¼ teaspoon Minor's Roasted Mirepoix Flavor Concentrate
1 teaspoon low-sodium ketchup

1. Prepare a 10-ounce, wide-mouth thermos by filling it with hot water.
2. Add the beef, potatoes, and carrots to a microwave-safe bowl; cover and microwave on high until heated through. Drain the hot water from the thermos and discard. Put the heated beef, potatoes, and carrots in the thermos.
3. Stir the Minor's bases and ketchup into the boiling water; pour over the ingredients in the thermos and stir. Seal the lid. At lunch, either stir the stew or shake the thermos a few times to combine the ingredients.

Luncheon Mozzarella Sandwich

Serves 1	
Per serving:	
Calories:	325.20
Protein:	11.87 g
Carbohydrates:	39.20 g
Total fat:	14.44 g
Sat. fat:	5.81 g
Cholesterol:	34.10 mg
Sodium:	198.28 mg
Fiber:	4.32 g

1 (1-ounce) slice whole-milk mozzarella cheese
2 (1-ounce) slices Old-Style Whole-Wheat Bread (page 215)
2 large iceberg lettuce leaves
2 teaspoons Homemade Mayonnaise (page 257)

2 wedges Oven-Dried Seasoned Tomatoes (page 194), finely chopped
1 scallion, white and green parts finely chopped
1 tablespoon finely minced celery
Pinch freshly ground black pepper

1. Place the mozzarella cheese between the slices of bread; store inside a sealable plastic bag or wrap in plastic wrap.
2. Wrap the cleaned lettuce leaves in a damp paper towel and store in another sealable plastic bag or wrap in plastic wrap.
3. Add the mayonnaise, tomatoes, scallion, celery, and pepper to a small plastic container; cover and keep sealed until ready to assemble the sandwich.
4. To assemble the sandwich, remove the top slice of bread and spread the mayonnaise mixture over the top of the mozzarella cheese slice. Top with the lettuce leaves. Place the top slice of bread back over the fillings; slice into wedges, if desired, and serve immediately.

❋ Keep It Crisp
Wrapping cleaned fresh greens (that have been dried in a salad spinner) in damp paper towels and then storing them inside a plastic bag will keep them crisp. They'll stay fresh for several days if kept in the vegetable crisper.

Chicken Salad Pita

1 serving Chicken Salad Mold
(page 15)

4 large iceberg lettuce leaves
1 small, whole-wheat pita

Place the chicken salad mold and lettuce leaves in 1 sealable plastic bag and the pita in another. To assemble the sandwich, flake the mold and mix together with the lettuce leaves, torn into bite-size pieces. Cut the pita in half and stuff with the chicken salad mixture.

❀ Pita Picks
The nutritional analysis for this recipe assumes that a regular, commercial whole-wheat pita was used; the sodium content will be lower if you use a reduced-sodium pita.

Serves 1	
Per serving:	
Calories:	190.68
Protein:	14.35 g
Carbohydrates:	20.02 g
Total fat:	6.47 g
Sat. fat:	2.13 g
Cholesterol:	58.50 mg
Sodium:	415.36 mg
Fiber:	3.40 g

Fruit Cup with Creamy Dressing

⅛ cup peeled and grated carrots
1 tablespoon raisins
¼ cup cubed or sliced apple
6 seedless red or green grapes
4 ounces plain nonfat yogurt
1 tablespoon unsweetened, no-salt-added applesauce

1 teaspoon lemon juice
¼ teaspoon honey
⅛ teaspoon Pumpkin Pie Spice (page 275)
⅛ teaspoon finely grated fresh lemon zest

Arrange the carrots and fruit in a dessert cup. Mix the yogurt, applesauce, lemon juice, honey, and Pumpkin Pie Spice together and drizzle over the fruit. Sprinkle lemon zest over the top.

Serves 1	
Per serving:	
Calories:	145.45
Protein:	7.20 g
Carbohydrates:	29.75 g
Total fat:	0.56 g
Sat. fat:	0.22 g
Cholesterol:	2.26 mg
Sodium:	94.48 mg
Fiber:	1.86 g

Spiced Mixed Nut Butter Crunchies

Serves 1	
Per serving:	
Calories:	273.57
Protein:	6.14 g
Carbohydrates:	54.29 g
Total fat:	6.92 g
Sat. fat:	0.97 g
Cholesterol:	0.00 mg
Sodium:	227.05 mg
Fiber:	9.12 g

2 tablespoons Spiced Mixed Nut
    Butter (page 265)
1 small banana, mashed

⅛ cup seedless raisins
4 large stalks celery

In a small bowl, mix together the Spiced Mixed Nut Butter, banana, and raisins. Evenly spread over the celery sticks.

❈ No Fridge at Work?

It's important to keep foods chilled to keep bacteria at bay. If you don't have a refrigerator at work, put your lunch foods in the freezer for 1 hour or overnight. That way your food will remain chilled, but be thawed by lunchtime.

APPENDIX A
Spice Blends

Herbal and Other Seasoning Mixtures

Using herbs is a delicious way to season dishes and to cut down on the amount of salt needed for flavor, too. Dried herb mixtures can be prepared in advance and stored in an airtight container. Dried spices and herbs tend to lose flavor the longer they're stored, so the age of your seasoning mixes can directly affect the amount you should add to a recipe. Grinding them can help revive the potency because it releases their essential oils; for that reason, wait to grind spices until just before you need them.

To grind the spices and dried herbs in seasoning blends, a spice grinder or mortar and pestle works best. Alternatively, you can use a small food processor (such as the Cuisinart Mini-Prep Plus mentioned in Appendix B) or a blender. Unless advised otherwise by a recipe, process a seasoning blend until it is crushed and coarsely ground.

Cajun Spice Blend

2 tablespoons paprika
1½ tablespoons garlic powder
1 tablespoon onion powder
½ tablespoon black pepper
2 teaspoons cayenne pepper
2 teaspoons dried oregano
2 teaspoons dried thyme

Middle Eastern Spice Blend

1 tablespoon ground coriander
1 tablespoon ground cumin
1 tablespoon turmeric
1 teaspoon ground cinnamon
1 teaspoon crushed dried mint

Old Bay Seasoning

1 tablespoon celery seeds
1 tablespoon whole black peppercorns
6 bay leaves
½ teaspoon whole cardamom
½ teaspoon mustard seeds
4 whole cloves
1 teaspoon sweet Hungarian paprika
¼ teaspoon mace

Pacific Rim

1 tablespoon Chinese 5-spice powder
1 tablespoon paprika
1 tablespoon ground dried ginger
1 teaspoon black pepper

Pasta Blend
5 tablespoons dried basil
3 tablespoons dried oregano
2 tablespoons dried thyme
1 teaspoon garlic powder

Poultry Seasoning
2 tablespoons dried basil
2 teaspoons dried rosemary
2 teaspoons dried marjoram
1 teaspoon dried thyme
1 teaspoon dried oregano
½ teaspoon dried sage
¼ teaspoon mustard powder
¼ teaspoon dried lemon granules, crushed

Pumpkin Pie Spice
4 teaspoons ground cinnamon
2 teaspoons ground dried ginger
½ teaspoon ground allspice
½ teaspoon ground cloves
1 teaspoon ground nutmeg

Sonoran Spice Blend
1 tablespoon ground chili powder
1 tablespoon black pepper
1 tablespoon crushed dried oregano
1 tablespoon crushed dried thyme
1 tablespoon crushed dried coriander
1 tablespoon garlic powder

Stuffing Blend
2 tablespoons dried rubbed sage
1 tablespoon dried sweet marjoram
2 teaspoons dried parsley
1¼ teaspoons dried celery flakes

Texas Seasoning
3 tablespoons dried cilantro
2 tablespoons dried oregano
4 teaspoons dried thyme
2 tablespoons salt-free chili powder
2 tablespoons freshly ground black pepper
2 tablespoons ground cumin
2 small crushed dried chili peppers
1 teaspoon garlic powder

Caribbean Spice Blend
1 tablespoon curry powder
1 tablespoon ground cumin
1 tablespoon ground allspice
1 tablespoon ground dried ginger
1 teaspoon ground cayenne pepper

Country Table Spice Blend
5 teaspoons dried thyme
4 teaspoons dried basil
4 teaspoons dried chervil
4 teaspoons dried tarragon

English Spice Blend

1 tablespoon juniper berries, crushed
1 tablespoon dried thyme
1 teaspoon black pepper
1 teaspoon ground cloves
1 tablespoon onion powder

Fines Herbes

3 tablespoons dried parsley
2 teaspoons dried chervil
2 teaspoons dried chives
1½ teaspoons dried tarragon

Fish and Seafood Herbs

5 teaspoons dried basil
5 teaspoons fennel seeds, crushed
4 teaspoons dried parsley
1 teaspoon dried lemon granules, crushed

French Spice Blend

1 tablespoon crushed dried tarragon
1 tablespoon crushed dried chervil
1 tablespoon onion powder

Italian Spice Blend

1 tablespoon dried basil
1 tablespoon dried thyme
1 tablespoon dried oregano
2 tablespoons garlic powder

Herbes de Provence

4 teaspoons dried oregano
2 teaspoons dried basil
2 teaspoons dried sweet marjoram
2 teaspoons dried thyme
1 teaspoon dried mint
1 teaspoon dried rosemary
1 teaspoon dried sage leaves
1 teaspoon fennel seeds, crushed
1 teaspoon dried lavender

Blackened Catfish Spice Blend

1 tablespoon sweet paprika
1 tablespoon garlic powder
1 tablespoon onion powder
2 teaspoons cayenne
2 teaspoons cracked black pepper
2 bay leaves, ground
1 teaspoon ground white pepper
1 teaspoon brown sugar
1 teaspoon mustard powder
1 teaspoon dried lemon granules, crushed
½ teaspoon dried thyme
¼ teaspoon dried oregano
¼ teaspoon ground cloves
Optional: 1 tablespoon hot paprika

Chipotle Chili Powder Spice Blend

2 tablespoons ground chipotle
1 tablespoon onion powder
1 tablespoon garlic powder
1 teaspoon unsweetened cocoa powder
½ teaspoon dried Mexican oregano
¼ teaspoon cayenne
¼ teaspoon ground cumin
¼ teaspoon ground cinnamon
⅛ teaspoon ground cloves
⅛ teaspoon dried mustard powder
Pinch dried lemon granules, crushed

Hot Curry Spice Blend

½ tablespoon ground coriander
½ tablespoon ground cumin
½ tablespoon turmeric
1 teaspoon salt-free chili powder
1 teaspoon ground dried ginger
1 teaspoon ground black pepper
½ teaspoon ground cardamom
½ teaspoon mustard powder
¼ teaspoon cayenne
¼ teaspoon ground cloves
⅛ teaspoon ground nutmeg
⅛ teaspoon ground cinnamon
Pinch saffron

Garam Masala Spice Blend

1 tablespoon ground coriander
2 teaspoons ground cardamom
1 teaspoon cracked black pepper
1 teaspoon ground cinnamon
1 teaspoon charnushka
1 teaspoon caraway seeds
½ teaspoon ground cloves
½ teaspoon freshly ground
China Number One ginger
¼ teaspoon ground nutmeg

Greek Spice Blend

1 tablespoon garlic powder
1 tablespoon dried mint
1 teaspoon dried dill (dill weed)
1 teaspoon freeze-dried chives
½ teaspoon ground cinnamon
½ teaspoon dried oregano
¼ teaspoon ground nutmeg
⅛ teaspoon cayenne

Bouquets Garnis

Leafy part of 1–2 celery stalks
2–3 sprigs fresh thyme
1 bay leaf
1 small bunch fresh parsley
1–2 sprigs fresh marjoram or oregano

Jerk Spice Blend

1 tablespoon brown mustard seeds
1 tablespoon onion powder
2 teaspoons ground dried ginger
2 teaspoons garlic powder
1 teaspoon ground allspice
1 teaspoon hot paprika
½ teaspoon dried thyme
½ teaspoon fennel seeds
½ teaspoon ground black pepper
¼ teaspoon cayenne
¼ teaspoon ground cloves

Citrus Pepper

1 tablespoon cracked or freshly
    ground black pepper
1 teaspoon dried orange granules, crushed
½ teaspoon dried lemon granules, crushed
½ teaspoon dried mint
½ teaspoon ground dried ginger
¼ teaspoon dried lime granules, crushed
¼ teaspoon ground cardamom
¼ teaspoon garlic powder
¼ teaspoon ground coriander
2 drops orange oil
Pinch cayenne

Sources and Suppliers

Equipment

BEST MANUFACTURERS
✍ *www.bestmfrs.com*
Sells baking stones, whisks, spatulas

CHAR-BROIL
✍ *www.charbroil.com*
Sells multiburner electric and gas grills (that allow for indirect grilling)

CHICAGO METALLIC
✍ *www.bakingpans.com*
Professional, Betty Crocker, and other baking pans

CUISINART
✍ *www.cuisinart.com*
3½-quart nonstick stainless (the pan referred to as "ovenproof large, deep nonstick sauté pan" throughout the book)
Coffee grinder (for grinding spices)
Convection Oven-Toaster-Broiler with Exact Heat Sensor
ICE-20 Automatic Frozen Yogurt–Ice Cream and Sorbet Maker
ICE-40BK Flavor Duo Frozen Yogurt–Ice Cream and Sorbet Maker
Mini-Prep Plus
PowerPrep Plus
SmartPower Premier 600-Watt Blender
Turbo Convection Steamer

DEMARLE INC, USA
✍ *www.DemarleUSA.com*
Silpat nonstick pan liners

KAISER BAKEWARE
✍ *www.kaiserbakeware.com*
Professional baking pans, springform pans, reusable parchment paper

LE CREUSET
Le Creuset of America
✍ *www.lecreuset.com*
Ovenproof nonstick skillets

MICROPLANE ZESTER
✍ *www.microplane.com*

PLEASANT HILL GRAINS
✍ *www.pleasanthillgrain.com*
Bamix Deluxe Hand Mixer (immersion blender)
Bosch Concept 7 Mixer
Bosch Small Coffee and Spice Mill
Bosch Universal Mixer
Kuhn Rikon (3.5-liter) Duromatic Pressure Cooker
Maverick MM1886 Grinder
Tilia Pro II Vacuum Food Saver
Zojirushi Bread Maker

TILIA
✍ *www.tilia.com*
FoodSaver (vacuum food-storage system)

WORLD KITCHEN, INC.

✐ *www.worldkitchen.com*

  Baker's Secret (dry measuring cups, measuring
    spoons)
  Chicago Cutlery
  Corningware (microwave- and ovenproof
    baking dishes)
  Oxo (kitchen gadgets: salad spinner, garlic
    press, Grind It hand spice grinders)
  Pyrex (liquid measuring cups, microwave- and
    ovenproof casseroles and other baking
    dishes)

Low-Sodium and No-Salt-Added Products

Advantage International Foods Corporation
✐ *www.advantagefoods.com*

American Spoon and American Spoon Foods
✐ *www.spoon.com*

Barry Farm
✐ *www.barryfarm.com*

Bragg Live Foods, Inc.
✐ *www.bragg.com*

CaJohns Fiery Foods
✐ *www.cajohns.com*

Cantisano Foods, Inc.
✐ *www.francescorinaldi.com*

Cascadian Farms
✐ *www.cascadianfarm.com*

Chicken of the Sea International
✐ *www.chickenofthesea.com*

Earth's Best Baby Foods
✐ *www.earthsbest.com*

Eden Foods, Inc.
✐ *www.edenfoods.com*

Del Monte
✐ *www.delmonte.com*

Ener-G
✐ *www.ener-g.com*

Enrico's
✐ *www.enricos.com*

Erewhon
U.S. Mills, Inc.
✐ *www.usmillsinc.com*

Francesco Rinaldi
✐ *www.francescorinaldi.com*

Frontier National Brands
✐ *www.frontiercoop.com*

Gold Seal
✐ *www.canfisco.com*

Good Health Natural Foods, Inc.
✐ *www.goodhealthnaturalfoods.com*

H. J. Heinz Company
✐ *www.heinz.com*

Hodgson Mill
✎ *www.hodgsonmill.com*

Hunt's
✎ *www.hunts.com*

Kenyon's Grist Mill
✎ *www.kenyonsgristmill.com*

Lang Naturals
✎ *www.langnaturals.com*

Laura's Lean Beef
✎ *www.laurasleanbeef.com*

Mary Lu Seafood
✎ *www.maryluseafoods.com*

Michigan Farm Cheese Dairy
✎ *www.andrulischeese.com*

Miller's Cheese
✎ *www.koshercheese.com*

Minor's Bases and Flavor Concentrates
✎ *www.soupbase.com*

Mother's Mountain
✎ *www.mothersmountain.com*

Muir Glen
✎ *www.muirglen.com*

Newman's Own Organics
✎ *www.newmansownorganics.com*

Nutty Guys
✎ *www.nuttyguys.com*

Organic Valley
✎ *www.organicvalley.com*

Purity Foods
✎ *www.purityfoods.com*

RealSalt
Redmond Minerals, Inc.
✎ *www.realsalt.com*

Shiloh Farms
✎ *www.users.nwark.com/~shilohf/*

Smucker's
The J.M. Smucker Company
✎ *www.smuckers.com*

Spectrum Naturals
Spectrum Organic Products, Inc.
✎ *www.spectrumorganic.com*

'Tis Tasty
✎ *www.tistasty.com*

VivaLac, Inc.
✎ *www.wheylow.com*

Westbrae Natural
The Hain Celestial Group
✎ *www.westbrae.com*

Whey Low
✎ *www.wheylow.com*

Spices and Salt-Free Spice Blends

Frontier National Brands
✐ *www.frontiercoop.com*

Mrs. Dash
✐ *www.mrsdash.com*

The Spice House
✐ *www.thespicehouse.com*

The Spice Hunter
✐ *www.spicehunter.com*

Index

-sauced stir-fried cod and veggies, 106
steamed peppered chicken, 79
Peppers, chipotle
adobo sauce, 252
chili powder spice blend, 277
-poblano sauce, 253
remoulade, 252
sweet pickled relish, 246
Peppers, jalapeño
apricot and jalapeño-grilled lamb steaks, 125
pomegranate pizzazz sauce, 255
salad dressings, 45
Pickles, reduced-sodium dill, 256
Pineapple, in carrot cupcakes, 237
Pita, chicken salad, 271
Pizza, see Pasta and pizza
Pizza-flavored soy nuts, 232
Plum sauce, 260
Pomegranate pizzazz sauce, 255
Popcorn
about: seasoning of, 240
cinnamon-sweet, 233
microwave air-popped, 233
party mix, 234
Pork
baked tenderloin dinner, 155
barbecue sandwiches, 154
braised herb-seasoned chops, 122
chops and fruited veggies bake, 124
easy slow-cooked, 152
easy sweet-and-sour, 153
honey-grilled tenderloin, 120
indoor-grilled garlic sausage, 122
Italian casserole, 140
liverwurst, 135
loin dinner in adobo sauce, 147
oven beef stew, 37
paella, 102
palate pleasin' potpie, 141–142
pepped-up sandwiches, 153
and sauerkraut soup, 36
seasoned roast, 137
slow-roasted ribs, 123
south of the border sausage, 130
speedy jambalaya, 39
sweet and spicy kielbasa, 127
sweet pepper and fennel sausage, 130
warm salad, 154
Potato(es)
about: roasting with beef, 121
apple-potato pancakes, 61
baked potato soup, 27
broccoli and roasted potato soup, 269

garlic-roasted potatoes frittata, 66
oven-fried potato wedges, 177
potato water sourdough starter, 222
sausage and egg casserole, 63
warm broccoli and potato salad, 49
yogurt "gravy" chicken thighs, 84
Potpie, palate pleasin' pork, 141–142
Poultry, see Chicken; Turkey
Pretzels, commercial, 234
Prunes, in palate pleasin' pork potpie, 141–142
Pumpkin and ginger soup, 24
Pumpkin pie spice blend, 275
Quinoa
about, 192
and artichoke pilaf, 192
Raspberry and lemon steamed custard, 239
Ravioli, spinach in tomato mushroom sauce, 201
Relish, zesty corn, 43
Remoulade sauce, 251
Risotto
golden delicious, 178
mushroom, 167
Rosemary, 118
Russian dressing, 51

S

Saffron vinaigrette, 47
Sage, 264
Salads and salad dressings, 41–58
about: fat-free dressing, 52
Caesar salad, 56
candied walnut salad with pomegranate vinaigrette, 52
couscous in black olive–lemon vinaigrette, 170
crab Louis, 57
creamed chicken dressing, 53
grilled steak salad, 48
Italian dressing, 55
layered fruit and spinach salad, 46
marinated mushroom salad, 42
pear salad with fat-free raspberry vinaigrette, 47
roasted shallot vinaigrette, 44
Russian dressing, 51
saffron vinaigrette, 47
spiced tuna salad with toasted sesame vinaigrette, 50
tabouleh salad, 54
Thousand Island dressing, 51
tofu, oil, and vinegar dressing, 43
tuna-pasta salad, 207
vegetables in warm citrus vinaigrette, 186

veggie-fruit salad, 45
Waldorf salad, 54
warm broccoli and potato salad, 49
zesty corn relish, 43
Salmon
easy oven-roasted steaks, 115
microwave-poached, 99
scramble, 156
Salt
benefits of eating less, vii–viii
cooking tips, xi–xii
nutrition analysis, x–xi
processed foods and, 92
seasoning without, 90
sodium chloride, vii, ix
substitutes for, 27
Sauces
about: sugar in commercial, 132
cauliflower in ginger cheese sauce, 188
chipotle peppers in adobo sauce, 252
cranberry, with turkey patties, 132
minted bread sauce, 129
peach sauce, 261
plum sauce, 260
pork loin dinner in adobo sauce, 147
remoulade, 251
Sauerkraut and pork soup, 36
Sausage, see also Turkey sausage
south of the border sausage, 130
sweet pepper and fennel sausage, 130
Scallops
boiled seafood plates, 144
seafood in Thai-curry bean sauce, 112–113
triple ginger stir-fried scallops and vegetables, 103
Seafood and seafood entrées, 95–115
about: cooked weight, 113; cooking evenly, 109; fresh versus frozen, 115; nutrition, 98
baked breaded fish with lemon, 114
baked orange roughy in white wine, 97
baked red snapper almandine, 109
baked seasoned bread crumb–crusted fish, 105
boiled seafood plates, 144
chili-sauced stir-fried cod and veggies, 106
citrus pepper orange roughy, 108
easy-baked cod, 108
easy oven-roasted salmon steaks, 115
fish and seafood herbs, 276
he-man serving-size gumbo, 20
Italian-seasoned baked fish, 111
microwaved-poached salmon, 99
orange roughy with Italian roasted vegetables, 101

THE EVERYTHING SERIES!

BUSINESS & PERSONAL FINANCE

Everything® Accounting Book
Everything® Budgeting Book, 2nd Ed.
Everything® Business Planning Book
Everything® Coaching and Mentoring Book, 2nd Ed.
Everything® Fundraising Book
Everything® Get Out of Debt Book
Everything® Grant Writing Book, 2nd Ed.
Everything® Guide to Buying Foreclosures
Everything® Guide to Fundraising, $15.95
Everything® Guide to Mortgages
Everything® Guide to Personal Finance for Single Mothers
Everything® Home-Based Business Book, 2nd Ed.
Everything® Homebuying Book, 3rd Ed., $15.95
Everything® Homeselling Book, 2nd Ed.
Everything® Human Resource Management Book
Everything® Improve Your Credit Book
Everything® Investing Book, 2nd Ed.
Everything® Landlording Book
Everything® Leadership Book, 2nd Ed.
Everything® Managing People Book, 2nd Ed.
Everything® Negotiating Book
Everything® Online Auctions Book
Everything® Online Business Book
Everything® Personal Finance Book
Everything® Personal Finance in Your 20s & 30s Book, 2nd Ed.
Everything® Personal Finance in Your 40s & 50s Book, $15.95
Everything® Project Management Book, 2nd Ed.
Everything® Real Estate Investing Book
Everything® Retirement Planning Book
Everything® Robert's Rules Book, $7.95
Everything® Selling Book
Everything® Start Your Own Business Book, 2nd Ed.
Everything® Wills & Estate Planning Book

COOKING

Everything® Barbecue Cookbook
Everything® Bartender's Book, 2nd Ed., $9.95
Everything® Calorie Counting Cookbook
Everything® Cheese Book
Everything® Chinese Cookbook
Everything® Classic Recipes Book
Everything® Cocktail Parties & Drinks Book
Everything® College Cookbook
Everything® Cooking for Baby and Toddler Book
Everything® Diabetes Cookbook
Everything® Easy Gourmet Cookbook
Everything® Fondue Cookbook
Everything® Food Allergy Cookbook, $15.95
Everything® Fondue Party Book
Everything® Gluten-Free Cookbook
Everything® Glycemic Index Cookbook
Everything® Grilling Cookbook
Everything® Healthy Cooking for Parties Book, $15.95
Everything® Holiday Cookbook
Everything® Indian Cookbook
Everything® Lactose-Free Cookbook
Everything® Low-Cholesterol Cookbook

Everything® Low-Fat High-Flavor Cookbook, 2nd Ed., $15.95
Everything® Low-Salt Cookbook
Everything® Meals for a Month Cookbook
Everything® Meals on a Budget Cookbook
Everything® Mediterranean Cookbook
Everything® Mexican Cookbook
Everything® No Trans Fat Cookbook
Everything® One-Pot Cookbook, 2nd Ed., $15.95
Everything® Organic Cooking for Baby & Toddler Book, $15.95
Everything® Pizza Cookbook
Everything® Quick Meals Cookbook, 2nd Ed., $15.95
Everything® Slow Cooker Cookbook
Everything® Slow Cooking for a Crowd Cookbook
Everything® Soup Cookbook
Everything® Stir-Fry Cookbook
Everything® Sugar-Free Cookbook
Everything® Tapas and Small Plates Cookbook
Everything® Tex-Mex Cookbook
Everything® Thai Cookbook
Everything® Vegetarian Cookbook
Everything® Whole-Grain, High-Fiber Cookbook
Everything® Wild Game Cookbook
Everything® Wine Book, 2nd Ed.

GAMES

Everything® 15-Minute Sudoku Book, $9.95
Everything® 30-Minute Sudoku Book, $9.95
Everything® Bible Crosswords Book, $9.95
Everything® Blackjack Strategy Book
Everything® Brain Strain Book, $9.95
Everything® Bridge Book
Everything® Card Games Book
Everything® Card Tricks Book, $9.95
Everything® Casino Gambling Book, 2nd Ed.
Everything® Chess Basics Book
Everything® Christmas Crosswords Book, $9.95
Everything® Craps Strategy Book
Everything® Crossword and Puzzle Book
Everything® Crosswords and Puzzles for Quote Lovers Book, $9.95
Everything® Crossword Challenge Book
Everything® Crosswords for the Beach Book, $9.95
Everything® Cryptic Crosswords Book, $9.95
Everything® Cryptograms Book, $9.95
Everything® Easy Crosswords Book
Everything® Easy Kakuro Book, $9.95
Everything® Easy Large-Print Crosswords Book
Everything® Games Book, 2nd Ed.
Everything® Giant Book of Crosswords
Everything® Giant Sudoku Book, $9.95
Everything® Giant Word Search Book
Everything® Kakuro Challenge Book, $9.95
Everything® Large-Print Crossword Challenge Book
Everything® Large-Print Crosswords Book
Everything® Large-Print Travel Crosswords Book
Everything® Lateral Thinking Puzzles Book, $9.95
Everything® Literary Crosswords Book, $9.95
Everything® Mazes Book
Everything® Memory Booster Puzzles Book, $9.95

Everything® Movie Crosswords Book, $9.95
Everything® Music Crosswords Book, $9.95
Everything® Online Poker Book
Everything® Pencil Puzzles Book, $9.95
Everything® Poker Strategy Book
Everything® Pool & Billiards Book
Everything® Puzzles for Commuters Book, $9.95
Everything® Puzzles for Dog Lovers Book, $9.95
Everything® Sports Crosswords Book, $9.95
Everything® Test Your IQ Book, $9.95
Everything® Texas Hold 'Em Book, $9.95
Everything® Travel Crosswords Book, $9.95
Everything® Travel Mazes Book, $9.95
Everything® Travel Word Search Book, $9.95
Everything® TV Crosswords Book, $9.95
Everything® Word Games Challenge Book
Everything® Word Scramble Book
Everything® Word Search Book

HEALTH

Everything® Alzheimer's Book
Everything® Diabetes Book
Everything® First Aid Book, $9.95
Everything® Green Living Book
Everything® Health Guide to Addiction and Recovery
Everything® Health Guide to Adult Bipolar Disorder
Everything® Health Guide to Arthritis
Everything® Health Guide to Controlling Anxiety
Everything® Health Guide to Depression
Everything® Health Guide to Diabetes, 2nd Ed.
Everything® Health Guide to Fibromyalgia
Everything® Health Guide to Menopause, 2nd Ed.
Everything® Health Guide to Migraines
Everything® Health Guide to Multiple Sclerosis
Everything® Health Guide to OCD
Everything® Health Guide to PMS
Everything® Health Guide to Postpartum Care
Everything® Health Guide to Thyroid Disease
Everything® Hypnosis Book
Everything® Low Cholesterol Book
Everything® Menopause Book
Everything® Nutrition Book
Everything® Reflexology Book
Everything® Stress Management Book
Everything® Superfoods Book, $15.95

HISTORY

Everything® American Government Book
Everything® American History Book, 2nd Ed.
Everything® American Revolution Book, $15.95
Everything® Civil War Book
Everything® Freemasons Book
Everything® Irish History & Heritage Book
Everything® World War II Book, 2nd Ed.

HOBBIES

Everything® Candlemaking Book
Everything® Cartooning Book
Everything® Coin Collecting Book
Everything® Digital Photography Book, 2nd Ed.

Everything® Drawing Book
Everything® Family Tree Book, 2nd Ed.
Everything® Guide to Online Genealogy, $15.95
Everything® Knitting Book
Everything® Knots Book
Everything® Photography Book
Everything® Quilting Book
Everything® Sewing Book
Everything® Soapmaking Book, 2nd Ed.
Everything® Woodworking Book

HOME IMPROVEMENT

Everything® Feng Shui Book
Everything® Feng Shui Decluttering Book, $9.95
Everything® Fix-It Book
Everything® Green Living Book
Everything® Home Decorating Book
Everything® Home Storage Solutions Book
Everything® Homebuilding Book
Everything® Organize Your Home Book, 2nd Ed.

KIDS' BOOKS

All titles are $7.95
Everything® Fairy Tales Book, $14.95
Everything® Kids' Animal Puzzle & Activity Book
Everything® Kids' Astronomy Book
Everything® Kids' Baseball Book, 5th Ed.
Everything® Kids' Bible Trivia Book
Everything® Kids' Bugs Book
Everything® Kids' Cars and Trucks Puzzle and Activity Book
Everything® Kids' Christmas Puzzle & Activity Book
Everything® Kids' Connect the Dots
  Puzzle and Activity Book
Everything® Kids' Cookbook, 2nd Ed.
Everything® Kids' Crazy Puzzles Book
Everything® Kids' Dinosaurs Book
Everything® Kids' Dragons Puzzle and Activity Book
Everything® Kids' Environment Book $7.95
Everything® Kids' Fairies Puzzle and Activity Book
Everything® Kids' First Spanish Puzzle and Activity Book
Everything® Kids' Football Book
Everything® Kids' Geography Book
Everything® Kids' Gross Cookbook
Everything® Kids' Gross Hidden Pictures Book
Everything® Kids' Gross Jokes Book
Everything® Kids' Gross Mazes Book
Everything® Kids' Gross Puzzle & Activity Book
Everything® Kids' Halloween Puzzle & Activity Book
Everything® Kids' Hanukkah Puzzle and Activity Book
Everything® Kids' Hidden Pictures Book
Everything® Kids' Horses Book
Everything® Kids' Joke Book
Everything® Kids' Knock Knock Book
Everything® Kids' Learning French Book
Everything® Kids' Learning Spanish Book
Everything® Kids' Magical Science Experiments Book
Everything® Kids' Math Puzzles Book
Everything® Kids' Mazes Book
Everything® Kids' Money Book, 2nd Ed.
Everything® Kids' Mummies, Pharaoh's, and Pyramids
  Puzzle and Activity Book
Everything® Kids' Nature Book
Everything® Kids' Pirates Puzzle and Activity Book
Everything® Kids' Presidents Book
Everything® Kids' Princess Puzzle and Activity Book
Everything® Kids' Puzzle Book

Everything® Kids' Racecars Puzzle and Activity Book
Everything® Kids' Riddles & Brain Teasers Book
Everything® Kids' Science Experiments Book
Everything® Kids' Sharks Book
Everything® Kids' Soccer Book
Everything® Kids' Spelling Book
Everything® Kids' Spies Puzzle and Activity Book
Everything® Kids' States Book
Everything® Kids' Travel Activity Book
Everything® Kids' Word Search Puzzle and Activity Book

LANGUAGE

Everything® Conversational Japanese Book with CD, $19.95
Everything® French Grammar Book
Everything® French Phrase Book, $9.95
Everything® French Verb Book, $9.95
Everything® German Phrase Book, $9.95
Everything® German Practice Book with CD, $19.95
Everything® Inglés Book
Everything® Intermediate Spanish Book with CD, $19.95
Everything® Italian Phrase Book, $9.95
Everything® Italian Practice Book with CD, $19.95
Everything® Learning Brazilian Portuguese Book with CD, $19.95
Everything® Learning French Book with CD, 2nd Ed., $19.95
Everything® Learning German Book
Everything® Learning Italian Book
Everything® Learning Latin Book
Everything® Learning Russian Book with CD, $19.95
Everything® Learning Spanish Book
Everything® Learning Spanish Book with CD, 2nd Ed., $19.95
Everything® Russian Practice Book with CD, $19.95
Everything® Sign Language Book, $15.95
Everything® Spanish Grammar Book
Everything® Spanish Phrase Book, $9.95
Everything® Spanish Practice Book with CD, $19.95
Everything® Spanish Verb Book, $9.95
Everything® Speaking Mandarin Chinese Book with CD, $19.95

MUSIC

Everything® Bass Guitar Book with CD, $19.95
Everything® Drums Book with CD, $19.95
Everything® Guitar Book with CD, 2nd Ed., $19.95
Everything® Guitar Chords Book with CD, $19.95
Everything® Guitar Scales Book with CD, $19.95
Everything® Harmonica Book with CD, $15.95
Everything® Home Recording Book
Everything® Music Theory Book with CD, $19.95
Everything® Reading Music Book with CD, $19.95
Everything® Rock & Blues Guitar Book with CD, $19.95
Everything® Rock & Blues Piano Book with CD, $19.95
Everything® Rock Drums Book with CD, $19.95
Everything® Singing Book with CD, $19.95
Everything® Songwriting Book

NEW AGE

Everything® Astrology Book, 2nd Ed.
Everything® Birthday Personology Book
Everything® Celtic Wisdom Book, $15.95
Everything® Dreams Book, 2nd Ed.
Everything® Law of Attraction Book, $15.95
Everything® Love Signs Book, $9.95
Everything® Love Spells Book, $9.95
Everything® Palmistry Book
Everything® Psychic Book
Everything® Reiki Book

Everything® Sex Signs Book, $9.95
Everything® Spells & Charms Book, 2nd Ed.
Everything® Tarot Book, 2nd Ed.
Everything® Toltec Wisdom Book
Everything® Wicca & Witchcraft Book, 2nd Ed.

PARENTING

Everything® Baby Names Book, 2nd Ed.
Everything® Baby Shower Book, 2nd Ed.
Everything® Baby Sign Language Book with DVD
Everything® Baby's First Year Book
Everything® Birthing Book
Everything® Breastfeeding Book
Everything® Father-to-Be Book
Everything® Father's First Year Book
Everything® Get Ready for Baby Book, 2nd Ed.
Everything® Get Your Baby to Sleep Book, $9.95
Everything® Getting Pregnant Book
Everything® Guide to Pregnancy Over 35
Everything® Guide to Raising a One-Year-Old
Everything® Guide to Raising a Two-Year-Old
Everything® Guide to Raising Adolescent Boys
Everything® Guide to Raising Adolescent Girls
Everything® Mother's First Year Book
Everything® Parent's Guide to Childhood Illnesses
Everything® Parent's Guide to Children and Divorce
Everything® Parent's Guide to Children with ADD/ADHD
Everything® Parent's Guide to Children with Asperger's
  Syndrome
Everything® Parent's Guide to Children with Anxiety
Everything® Parent's Guide to Children with Asthma
Everything® Parent's Guide to Children with Autism
Everything® Parent's Guide to Children with Bipolar Disorder
Everything® Parent's Guide to Children with Depression
Everything® Parent's Guide to Children with Dyslexia
Everything® Parent's Guide to Children with Juvenile Diabetes
Everything® Parent's Guide to Children with OCD
Everything® Parent's Guide to Positive Discipline
Everything® Parent's Guide to Raising Boys
Everything® Parent's Guide to Raising Girls
Everything® Parent's Guide to Raising Siblings
Everything® Parent's Guide to Raising Your
  Adopted Child
Everything® Parent's Guide to Sensory Integration Disorder
Everything® Parent's Guide to Tantrums
Everything® Parent's Guide to the Strong-Willed Child
Everything® Parenting a Teenager Book
Everything® Potty Training Book, $9.95
Everything® Pregnancy Book, 3rd Ed.
Everything® Pregnancy Fitness Book
Everything® Pregnancy Nutrition Book
Everything® Pregnancy Organizer, 2nd Ed., $16.95
Everything® Toddler Activities Book
Everything® Toddler Book
Everything® Tween Book
Everything® Twins, Triplets, and More Book

PETS

Everything® Aquarium Book
Everything® Boxer Book
Everything® Cat Book, 2nd Ed.
Everything® Chihuahua Book
Everything® Cooking for Dogs Book
Everything® Dachshund Book
Everything® Dog Book, 2nd Ed.
Everything® Dog Grooming Book

Everything® Dog Obedience Book
Everything® Dog Owner's Organizer, $16.95
Everything® Dog Training and Tricks Book
Everything® German Shepherd Book
Everything® Golden Retriever Book
Everything® Horse Book, 2nd Ed., $15.95
Everything® Horse Care Book
Everything® Horseback Riding Book
Everything® Labrador Retriever Book
Everything® Poodle Book
Everything® Pug Book
Everything® Puppy Book
Everything® Small Dogs Book
Everything® Tropical Fish Book
Everything® Yorkshire Terrier Book

REFERENCE

Everything® American Presidents Book
Everything® Blogging Book
Everything® Build Your Vocabulary Book, $9.95
Everything® Car Care Book
Everything® Classical Mythology Book
Everything® Da Vinci Book
Everything® Einstein Book
Everything® Enneagram Book
Everything® Etiquette Book, 2nd Ed.
Everything® Family Christmas Book, $15.95
Everything® Guide to C. S. Lewis & Narnia
Everything® Guide to Divorce, 2nd Ed., $15.95
Everything® Guide to Edgar Allan Poe
Everything® Guide to Understanding Philosophy
Everything® Inventions and Patents Book
Everything® Jacqueline Kennedy Onassis Book
Everything® John F. Kennedy Book
Everything® Mafia Book
Everything® Martin Luther King Jr. Book
Everything® Pirates Book
Everything® Private Investigation Book
Everything® Psychology Book
Everything® Public Speaking Book, $9.95
Everything® Shakespeare Book, 2nd Ed.

RELIGION

Everything® Angels Book
Everything® Bible Book
Everything® Bible Study Book with CD, $19.95
Everything® Buddhism Book
Everything® Catholicism Book
Everything® Christianity Book
Everything® Gnostic Gospels Book
Everything® Hinduism Book, $15.95
Everything® History of the Bible Book
Everything® Jesus Book
Everything® Jewish History & Heritage Book
Everything® Judaism Book
Everything® Kabbalah Book
Everything® Koran Book
Everything® Mary Book
Everything® Mary Magdalene Book
Everything® Prayer Book

Everything® Saints Book, 2nd Ed.
Everything® Torah Book
Everything® Understanding Islam Book
Everything® Women of the Bible Book
Everything® World's Religions Book

SCHOOL & CAREERS

Everything® Career Tests Book
Everything® College Major Test Book
Everything® College Survival Book, 2nd Ed.
Everything® Cover Letter Book, 2nd Ed.
Everything® Filmmaking Book
Everything® Get-a-Job Book, 2nd Ed.
Everything® Guide to Being a Paralegal
Everything® Guide to Being a Personal Trainer
Everything® Guide to Being a Real Estate Agent
Everything® Guide to Being a Sales Rep
Everything® Guide to Being an Event Planner
Everything® Guide to Careers in Health Care
Everything® Guide to Careers in Law Enforcement
Everything® Guide to Government Jobs
Everything® Guide to Starting and Running a Catering Business
Everything® Guide to Starting and Running a Restaurant
Everything® Guide to Starting and Running a Retail Store
Everything® Job Interview Book, 2nd Ed.
Everything® New Nurse Book
Everything® New Teacher Book
Everything® Paying for College Book
Everything® Practice Interview Book
Everything® Resume Book, 3rd Ed.
Everything® Study Book

SELF-HELP

Everything® Body Language Book
Everything® Dating Book, 2nd Ed.
Everything® Great Sex Book
Everything® Guide to Caring for Aging Parents, $15.95
Everything® Self-Esteem Book
Everything® Self-Hypnosis Book, $9.95
Everything® Tantric Sex Book

SPORTS & FITNESS

Everything® Easy Fitness Book
Everything® Fishing Book
Everything® Guide to Weight Training, $15.95
Everything® Krav Maga for Fitness Book
Everything® Running Book, 2nd Ed.
Everything® Triathlon Training Book, $15.95

TRAVEL

Everything® Family Guide to Coastal Florida
Everything® Family Guide to Cruise Vacations
Everything® Family Guide to Hawaii
Everything® Family Guide to Las Vegas, 2nd Ed.
Everything® Family Guide to Mexico
Everything® Family Guide to New England, 2nd Ed.

Everything® Family Guide to New York City, 3rd Ed.
Everything® Family Guide to Northern California and Lake Tahoe
Everything® Family Guide to RV Travel & Campgrounds
Everything® Family Guide to the Caribbean
Everything® Family Guide to the Disneyland® Resort, California Adventure®, Universal Studios®, and the Anaheim Area, 2nd Ed.
Everything® Family Guide to the Walt Disney World Resort®, Universal Studios®, and Greater Orlando, 5th Ed.
Everything® Family Guide to Timeshares
Everything® Family Guide to Washington D.C., 2nd Ed.

WEDDINGS

Everything® Bachelorette Party Book, $9.95
Everything® Bridesmaid Book, $9.95
Everything® Destination Wedding Book
Everything® Father of the Bride Book, $9.95
Everything® Green Wedding Book, $15.95
Everything® Groom Book, $9.95
Everything® Jewish Wedding Book, 2nd Ed., $15.95
Everything® Mother of the Bride Book, $9.95
Everything® Outdoor Wedding Book
Everything® Wedding Book, 3rd Ed.
Everything® Wedding Checklist, $9.95
Everything® Wedding Etiquette Book, $9.95
Everything® Wedding Organizer, 2nd Ed., $16.95
Everything® Wedding Shower Book, $9.95
Everything® Wedding Vows Book, 3rd Ed., $9.95
Everything® Wedding Workout Book
Everything® Weddings on a Budget Book, 2nd Ed., $9.95

WRITING

Everything® Creative Writing Book
Everything® Get Published Book, 2nd Ed.
Everything® Grammar and Style Book, 2nd Ed.
Everything® Guide to Magazine Writing
Everything® Guide to Writing a Book Proposal
Everything® Guide to Writing a Novel
Everything® Guide to Writing Children's Books
Everything® Guide to Writing Copy
Everything® Guide to Writing Graphic Novels
Everything® Guide to Writing Research Papers
Everything® Guide to Writing a Romance Novel, $15.95
Everything® Improve Your Writing Book, 2nd Ed.
Everything® Writing Poetry Book